12/13/96

For my "dear" friends

Manny Lloyd and Robert White

with love

This Friday the thirteenth.

[illegible]

Life of a Country Doctor

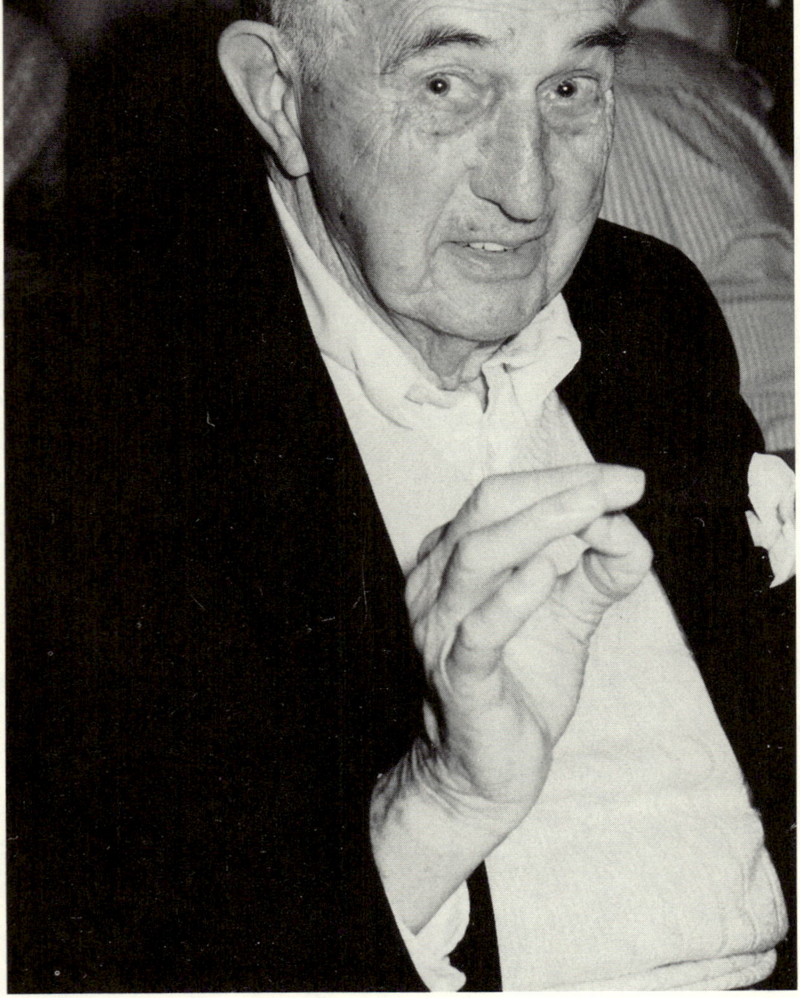

LIFE

OF A

COUNTRY DOCTOR

By James Edwards Cameron, M.D.

Edited by Edith Cameron Blankenship

Black Belt Press
Montgomery

The Black Belt Press
P.O. Box 551
Montgomery, AL 36101

 Published in the United States by the Black Belt Press, a division of the Black Belt Communications Group, Inc., Montgomery, Alabama.

Library of Congress Cataloging-in-Publication Data

Cameron, James Edwards, 1907-
Life of a country doctor / by James Edwards Cameron ; edited by Edith Cameron Blankenship.
p. cm.
Includes index.
ISBN 1-881320-57-x
1. Cameron, James Edwards, 1907- . 2. Physicians—Alabama—Biography. 3. Medicine, Rural—Alabama. I. Blankenship, Edith Cameron. II. Title.
R154.C235A3 1996
610' .92—dc20
[B] 96-23008
CIP

BOOK DESIGN BY RANDALL WILLIAMS

The Black Belt, defined by its dark, rich soil, stretches across central Alabama. It was the heart of the cotton belt. It was and is a place of great beauty, of extreme wealth and grinding poverty, of pain and joy. Here we take our stand, listening to the past, looking to the future.

Overleaf: *Dr. Jim Cameron —1988.*

Photographs on pages 2, 20, 23, 28, 36, 46, 48, 83, 84, 93, 95, 97, 98, 99, 104, 109, 111, 112, 113, 114, and 115 were provided by the Cameron Family.

TO EDITH

My bride of fifty-six years,
who has helped make this life as a country doctor
happy as well as rewarding

Contents

Life of a Country Doctor

Preface

When I was a very small child, I loved hearing Granny tell stories about my daddy as a little boy playing with Mason Loy, Freddie Sington, and others in their neighborhood. As I grew up, I learned more bits and pieces about his life and heard phrases such as "She's a fine woman, they say!" and "Mr. White, you don't know enough anatomy to pick a chicken." I also heard all my life of characters such as Dr. Justice, Wood Fuller, Brooks Forehand, and Dr. Harlan and of places such as Tulane, "the Corner," and Eclectic. And, of course, I was impressed by Daddy's stories about driving as a very young teenager and going to college at age fifteen.

I have also had many of Daddy's friends and fellow physicians tell me they enjoyed his stories of his early medical practice and other experiences. Many of them have encouraged me to get these stories on paper to preserve them.

In fact, the idea for this book grew out of a speech Daddy was asked to give to the Tallapoosa County Medical Society in 1991. When I typed that speech, I realized not only the historical importance of those anecdotes about medical practice in Tallapoosa County in the thirties, forties, and fifties but how much more he could have told.

Yet only when I began transcribing his tapes recounting his life did I realize how many of his stories I had not heard and how little I really knew about his early life and his family. I knew very little of my grandparents and even less about my great- grandparents. I'd never heard of Raydeen or of the pigeons stolen from the Catholic church. And if I, who have known him almost fifty-four years, didn't know these tales, certainly his other children, grandchildren, great-grandchildren and friends would not know them either.

Thus off and on over a period of four years, he has taped and I have transcribed, ordered, and edited the reminiscences which make up his life, the life of a country doctor. Certainly to those of us in the family he is much more than a doctor—he is husband, father, and grandfather. He is Boompa, and this is his story.

EDITH CAMERON BLANKENSHIP

INTRODUCTION

My life span so far has gone from one end of the twentieth century to the other, minus a few years on each end. And this has been a century of unparalleled change and progress. In 1903 man first devised a steerable airplane; later in this same century a man and woman flew non-stop around the world with very little hoopla attached to their achievement. Electronic devices have also advanced from very elementary communication by Morse code to satellite distribution of color television between planets. Ground transportation has gone from the earliest motorcars which crept along to present-day race cars that proceed at several hundred miles per hour.

During this same time period, medicine has advanced so that the killer diseases of the early twentieth century (tuberculosis, malaria, and typhoid) occur only rarely today, while cancer, heart disease and AIDS have risen to the top of the ranks as killers. Whereas when I was born, life expectancy was approximately fifty years, today it is more than seventy years, and it is not at all unusual to encounter centenarians.

When I began medical practice in the 1930s, ninety percent of doctors were general practitioners. Now at least ninety percent are specialists, and few, if any, of the family practitioners (today's closest equivalent to the general practitioner) make house calls as practically all doctors did then. Instead of the country doctor doing everything from removing an injured eye to treating babies with club feet or performing Caesarean sections, now the family doctor does very little, if any, surgery—certainly no major surgery even when confronted by the extreme need for such.

I performed operations of many kinds during my years of practice and stopped doing them when better-qualified doctors became available. This same principle held true for obstetrics. After delivering about twenty-five hundred babies, I retired from that field at about age sixty.

In the thirties most diagnoses were arrived at by the doctor's own visual, auditory, and tactile senses. In the last fifty years mechanical and electronic devices as well as laboratory tests have become much more frequently used in determining a patient's condition.

Another drastic change which I have witnessed in medicine concerns financial consideration. During the Depression of 1929–1935, some doctors were paid in species other than money. In fact, the biggest fee I ever collected was a school bus full of corn in payment for extensive surgery. In those days when some people were without jobs and had practically no income, a hard-working general practitioner struggled for the necessities of life himself. Today many surgical procedures require pre-payment or guarantee of payment by a third party, *i.e.*, an insurance company. Furthermore, though only a few years ago the by-laws of the state medical association forbade discussion at meetings of monetary matters, today money is the chief item on the agenda.

Perhaps we should ask ourselves if this is really progress.

Many people have had a good influence on my behavior and learning. I shall try to name some of them, but their importance in my life should not be judged by the order in which they are listed. Certainly Granny Edwards, my grandmother by adoption, was a strong personality who had a predominating influence in the first thirty-three years of my life. Others who were important in the molding of my career were my step-father, George G. Menefee; R. H. Whorton, who loaned me money to finish school; Dr. George T. Pack, the most outstanding teacher I ever studied under; Dr. Lloyd Noland, who not only taught me but loaned me money when I was ill; Dr. Earl Conwell, who taught me many orthopedic procedures during my internship; Dr. Hartwell Cocke, who treated me when I had tuberculosis; Dr. Adrian Taylor, an outstanding surgeon whom I followed for a few months; and Dr. Seale Harris, who was responsible for my going into practice in central Alabama.

Finally, the person who has been most influential in my life for the past fifty-six plus years has been my wife, Edith. Being the wife of a country general practitioner is trying to say the least. My wife has had to suffer from frequent interruptions of both meals and sleep and endured an often-absent husband who could never be counted on to babysit for his own children. Through all these years, Edith has been not only supportive of my efforts but most generous in her praise of my activities.

These reminiscences of an old man are being set down at the insistence of my wife and children. They think that perhaps they and others will at some time be interested in hearing about the life of their husband and father, my life as a country doctor.

James E. Cameron, M.D.

Life of a Country Doctor

1

Tuberculosis, Mom, and Stealing Pigeons

MY NAME IS JAMES EDWARDS CAMERON, AND I was born on August 18, 1907, in Birmingham, Alabama. My parents were Hallie James Edwards and William James Cameron, Jr. My mother was born in Richmond, Kentucky, on April 17, 1886, to a Mr. and Mrs. James. Some years later, after her mother had died (whether in childbirth or later, I am not sure), her father gave his daughter up for adoption to his friends Frank and Virginia Edwards of Birmingham. My father was the son of William James and Mary Elizabeth Smith Cameron; their fourth child, he was born in the very young town of Birmingham, Alabama, on July 21, 1881. (His older siblings were Smith, Pauline, and Andrew Cameron.) His mother died only two weeks later, and my grandfather remarried in 1883. By his second wife, Mary Ward Cameron, he had three more children (George, Mary, and Margaret). Thus my father had several half and whole brothers and sisters; however, the only ones whom I ever knew well were Uncle Andy and Aunt Pauline, who incidentally lived well into her nineties. Uncle Andy, although a diabetic and alcoholic, was a prominent surgeon who had his office in the middle of Birmingham. He served as surgeon for the L & N Railroad and Liberty National Life Insurance Company which was practically brand new at the time. Most of the stock in Liberty National was then held by the Samford family. Later Frank Spain, an attorney in Birmingham, became an important stock holder in the company by taking stock as pay for his legal services to this young

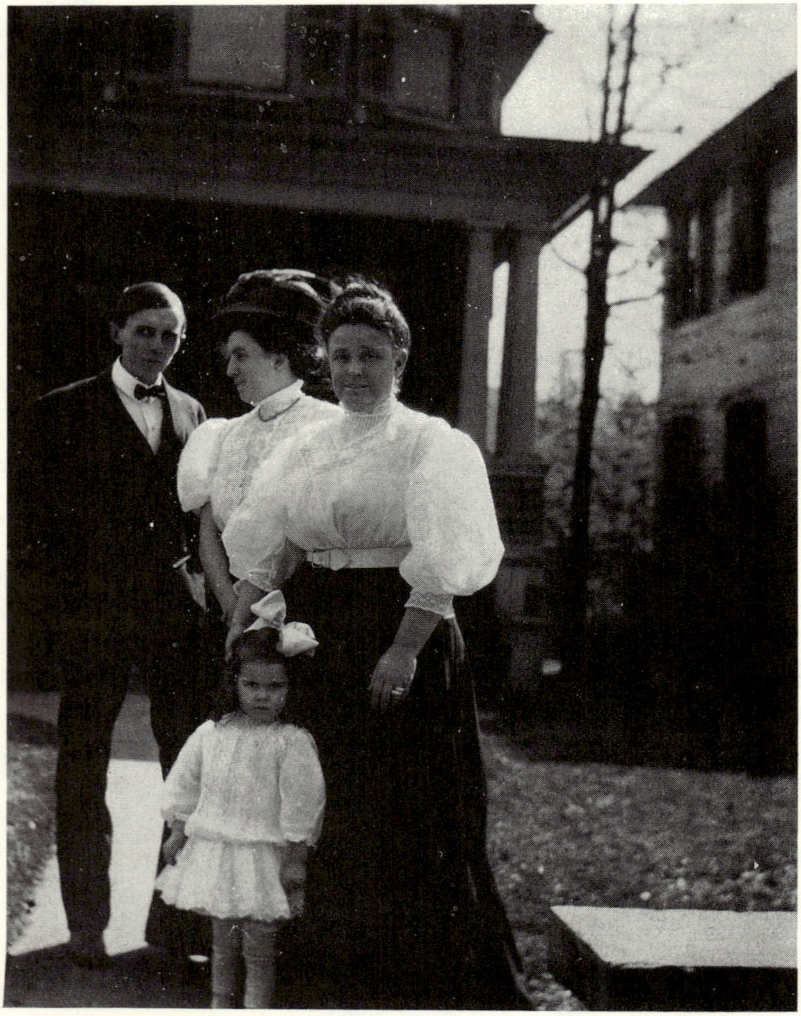

Will, Hallie, and Virginia Cameron with Jennie Edwards (in 1907) in front of house where Jim Cameron was born.

company. Thus Mr. Spain became immensely wealthy. Though I was no kin to the Spains, my father's half sister, Margaret Cameron, married Frank Spain. Their daughter Peggy (wife of Billy McDonald) is also still living. [*See* "Ancestor Report for James Edwards Cameron" and "Descendant Report for William James Cameron" in the Appendix.]

There are very few people who live to be eighty plus who have been governed by anything as small as the tubercle bacillus all of their lives, even before the life began; however, it has been my fate to have had such experience with the disease tuberculosis. To put the thing in perspective, we must recognize that many people died of tuberculosis when I was a child. The bacillus had been discovered by a German scientist only about forty years before I was born. And it had been studied and cultured by Koch only seven or eight years before my birth. People dreaded consumption or tuberculosis because it was a great killer and no respecter of persons. The statistics of the world show that few diseases were greater killers at the time.

In my own family, my mother's father, Frank Edwards, had acquired tuberculosis somewhere, and he passed it on to his adopted child. They were both sick with tuberculosis during the early part of this century. Mr. Edwards lived on until 1913 and my mother until 1922, but their lives were greatly influenced by this disease for which there was no effective treatment in those days. People sought help from the disease by going to a dry climate, eating a large amount of food, and resting. There was nothing else which could be done, no medicines which could help at all. The chest Xray was not invented until about 1904. Thus the treatment was to isolate people with this disease from the general population, burn their sputum to keep down contagion, and treat them as people who were unable to work. Some people with the disease did continue to work and lived on for years while others were killed very rapidly by it.

My mother found that she had tuberculosis about the time that my sister Virginia was born in 1905. Naturally, she was greatly concerned about her health when she found that she was pregnant with another child two years later. There was mixed opinion at that time about whether the woman with tuberculosis should be aborted; some thought a pregnancy was dangerous while others thought it might even increase the woman's chances of getting well. And some people even then did get well from tuberculosis. In fact, it was probably the most curable of the chronic diseases. People did not get well of rheumatoid arthritis, diabetes, chronic kidney disease, or chronic liver disease. But the knowledge that some did recover from tuberculosis was the thought my mother had when I was born in 1907.

Soon after I was born, my mother weaned me in the hope that she would not transfer the disease to me through her milk. At that time she was taken to Denver, Colorado, and there in the high dry climate of Denver, it was hoped that she and my grandfather would recover. They and I lived out there for a year or two. Mother had remissions of the disease, but Mr. Edwards apparently went downhill fairly rapidly. In 1913, he finally died of the disease, after having been in various sanitaria.

My mother had studied the piano at the Juilliard School of Music in New York about 1900. During her periodic remissions from tuberculosis she was able to sell pianos for the Forbes Piano Company and to play the piano professionally and lead an active social life. My mother and father were divorced in 1910 or 1911. My sister and I were taken over by my mother's mother by adoption, Granny Edwards, because Mother was trying to get well. She spent some time in sanataria in Saranac Lake, New York, and in Asheville, North Carolina. She was back and forth, disabled and able for a good many years. Finally she met Mr. George G. Menefee during one of the times she was in remission and apparently doing very well. They married in 1914 and moved to Syracuse, New York, leaving Virginia and me with Granny in Birmingham. Apparently my mother did very well up there. They came back to Birmingham, but soon afterward my mother had another episode with tuberculosis. During all these years, Virginia and I were cared for by a loving grandmother, and she was that.

Granny, or Mom as we called her, was a short, stout woman who was strict in her discipline of Virginia and me. She always called me "James" though my sister and friends called me "Jimmy." And though she spoke politely, we knew her commands for what they were. For instance, she often told me, "James, you may wash the dishes!" And I knew that I not only "might" but had better do it.

One day when I was undoubtedly feeling my oats, Granny said if I didn't do such and such she would pop my jaws. I replied, "Well, pop away, Old Lady." She did and nearly knocked me in a flip. And to this day I remember exactly what part of the house I was in and how well she did strike me. She used to say, "I never struck you a blow amiss, except when I struck at you and missed." And that was about the way it was.

One night we had a Mr. J. P. Glass as a guest for dinner. He was a suitor to a nurse who boarded at our house. When the meal was practically over, the servant passed around an assortment of French pastries. When they came to me, I shook my head in refusal and said, "Thank you, I don't care for one."

Immediately, either Granny or my mother said, "James, we thought you were especially fond of chocolate eclair."

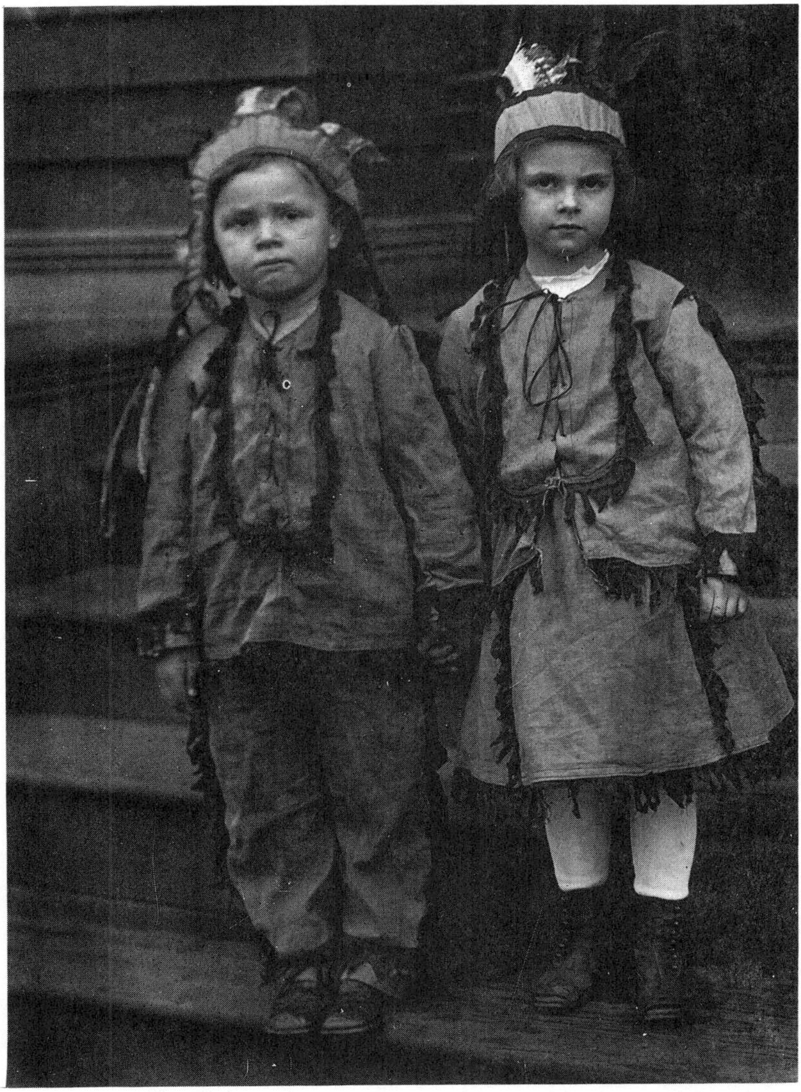

Jim Cameron and his sister Virginia in Indian costumes— ca. 1910.

I answered, "Yes, I like chocolate eclair, but Mr. Glass got the one I wanted."

Granny replied, "You may leave the table and finish your supper in the kitchen with the servants. You don't deserve to eat in here with us!"

One of my very earliest memories was of seeing an enormous fire in New York City. For some reason, Granny, Mother, Virginia, and I were in New York at the time. I remember Granny taking Virginia and me out on a ferry into the middle of the Hudson River where we watched this huge fire. And, although I was only three or four years old at the time, I remember that the fire trucks were mostly horse-drawn (automobile engines were not reliable).

As a boy I was accident prone. First, I broke my nose in a tricycle accident. Another time I broke my clavicle in a twelve-foot fall from the back steps and my right arm in a vault over the bannisters. I had the usual childhood illnesses—measles, mumps, and whooping cough. Nearly all children had those diseases in those days; in fact, they were known as the ODC (ordinary diseases of childhood). I had an absess form in my axilla (armpit) which had to be incised, and I had a tonsilectomy when I was about seven years old. After the tonsilectomy, I got to ride home from the hospital in the first auto-powered ambulance in Birmingham, a Great Eagle owned by the Lige Loy Funeral Home. Mr. Loy, a so-called uncle, was not only our neighbor but the husband of Granny's sister Susie. But other than those incidents and the diseases of childhood, I remained remarkably well.

I was never a super athlete but tried awfully hard to play games. Despite Granny's efforts to make a lady of Virginia, she could always run or skate faster than I could. While I was never a great athlete, I could usually make the team whether it was in swimming, diving, basketball, football, or baseball. I was surrounded by boys who were fine athletes, and I could easily tell the difference. My body was long and thin; my muscles were stringy, not bunched at all. However, I did play baseball with my classmates on both the junior and senior teams. The teams were divided by weight with the boys weighing less than one hundred pounds making up the junior team and those of a hundred pounds or more making up the senior team. The ones who weighed less than one hundred pounds and were capable might play on both teams. I was lucky enough to play outfield on one team and catch on the other, so I did have some physical ability. I mention that not to brag but to show that I was not a sickly child though thin and wiry.

Among the boys I played with in the neighborhood as a child were Cecil Joseph Matthews, Mason Loy (the son of Lige and Susie Loy), and Fred Sington. Fred was a great big boy who was an only child. His mother insisted that Freddie wasn't fat, he was just muscular. Sure enough, he was muscular. He later won All-American recognition as a football player and played professional baseball with the Washington Senators. He was also a Phi Beta Kappa student.

Certainly I got into my share of mischief when I was a boy. For instance, Philip Shaw (who lived across the street) and I decided one day to get us some pigeons. We knew that the Catholic church in downtown Birmingham had plenty of pigeons in its belfry, so we rode the streetcar downtown, climbed up into the belfry, and filled our shirts with pigeons. Now in all that climbing around to catch the pigeons we got pretty dirty, so after we had captured our prey, we washed our hands in the very convenient basin of water we found in the church (the holy water). Then we boarded the streetcar again and took our pigeons home. We had built a cote for them, but as soon as we turned them into the cote, the pigeons took off and flew right back to the church.

The house in which I was born was one on the corner of Eleventh Avenue and Fourteenth Streets (1331 Eleventh Avenue South) belonging to my Edwards grandparents. We lived there until about the time I started to school; then Granny rented that house and we moved to a smaller house on Thirttieth Street South between upper Highland Avenue and lower Highland Avenue, and I attended Lakeview School for one year. Then we moved back to Eleventh Avenue, and since Ullman School was nearest to that house, I attended grammar school there. It was surrounded by black people and first generation Americans from Italy and Greece. Our principal was C. P. Underwood, a most marvelous man for all seasons. He taught us baseball, basketball, and gardening (during 1917–1918 we raised a garden on the school grounds). To be sent to Mr. Underwood's office was very bad; however, luckily when I was sent, he and I talked baseball.

In December 1917, when I was ten years old and Virginia was twelve, our father was living at a place called Battelle, Alabama, about two miles inside Alabama on Lookout Mountain. Just across the state line was the town of Rising Fawn, Georgia. An iron furnace had been built there, and coal and iron had been mined from the Lookout Mountain Range. The company my father worked for, the Crawford Vaughn Boiler and Locomotive Works, had contracted to dismantle this blast furnace, label the parts, and ship all to India to be reassembled there and used to make iron for the war effort. Virginia and I rode the train up to Battelle to spend a few days in the boarding house with Daddy. At that time the town had become a ghost town with hundreds of abandoned homes. The iron mines were off to the east of us, and we went up and saw where the mines had been. I still remember one incident which happened there. Much to my father's consternation and my sister's amazement, I climbed a steep rock cliff. If I had fallen, I would certainly have been killed, but obviously I didn't fall.

2

Cullam Street, Homebrew, and Waddell

About the time I finished grammar school, Pop (as we called our stepfather), Mother, Virginia, and I moved to a house on Cullam Street, on the south side of Birmingham. Here we had an apartment in the home of a Mrs. Snell. Mrs. Snell, a widow, was the movie inspector for the city of Birmingham. She was very straight-laced and strict in her views about what movies should be shown in Birmingham. As a result, the newspapers didn't like her very much. Once we had an ice storm, during which Mrs. Snell had a fall. *The Birmingham News* reported, "Mrs. Snell fell during the ice storm and hurt her somewhat."

Mrs. Snell's son Robert was a senior in high school, and I remember riding down to Tuscaloosa, a distance of sixty miles over unpaved roads, with Robert and his mother when they went to arrange for living quarters for him at the University of Alabama. One of the things I remember about this trip was that Tutwiler Hall was just being finished, and I think that was the first fall the university became co-educational.

During the year or so that we lived on Cullam Street, one of the friends with whom I played was Sammy Stern who lived down on the corner. Sammy's father had joined the Jewish country club, and one day Sammy and I walked from Cullam Street out to the country club where I used Sammy's clubs to play the first round of golf I ever played. Of course, we also walked back home, another couple of miles.

There was another family on that street named Angel. One of them

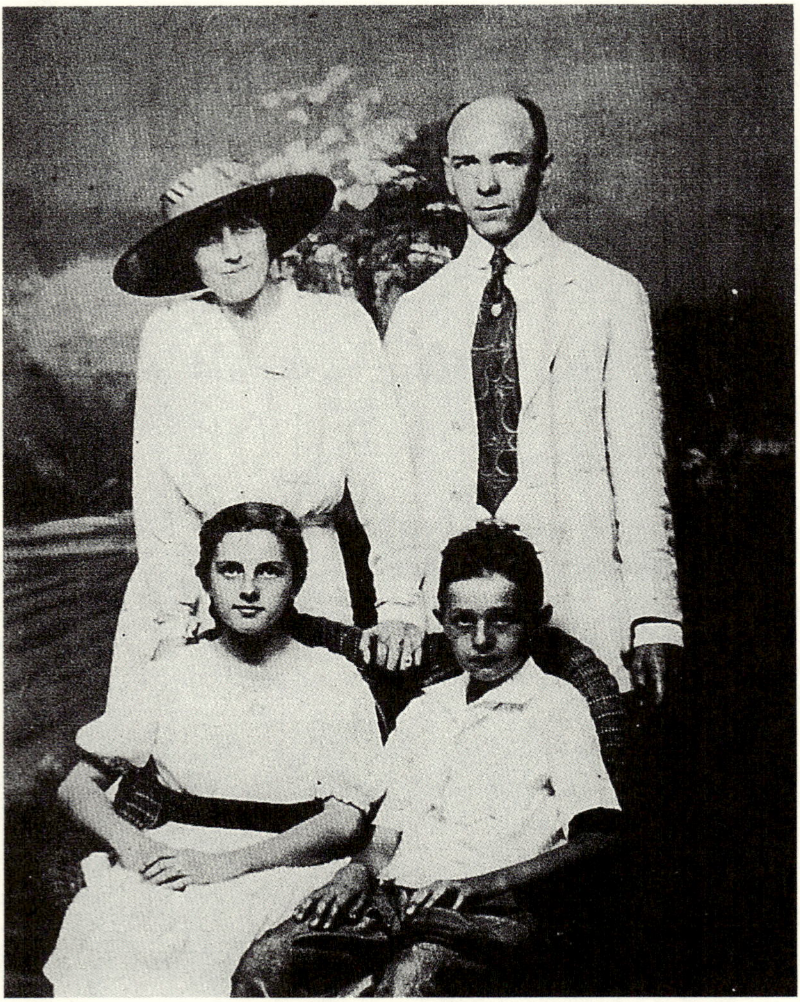

Hallie and George Menefee, Virginia and Jim Cameron—1916.

was named Rosser, but I don't remember the names of all the others. Another boy named Roy who lived in that neighborhood followed the dictates of the masses and got into all kinds of mischief. One of the things he did was to go up on nearby Red Mountain and take some blasting caps out of an abandoned mine. While he was playing with these blasting caps, one of them exploded and put out one of his eyes.

About two blocks away lived a family named Streit who had several boys and several girls. The youngest child of this family was Edward Morris "Buck" Streit who became a close friend of mine and remained a friend for many years.

A year or two later, Mother and Pop decided to buy a house on the edge of Birmingham in what is now Mountain Brook, so we children moved out there with them. Pop bought a cow and a few chickens so that Mother could have plenty of fresh milk and eggs which were believed to be conducive to the cure of tuberculosis. (Certainly nutrition is important, but I don't think eggs and milk are the answers to this disease.)

In our new neighborhood, one of our neighbors was an older brother of Buck's, Brice Streit. He had served in the First World War and was then in the real estate business with his father. He and his wife Marge were our closest neighbors though they lived a half mile from us. They were also our close friends of whom I have many fond memories.

Several years later an incident occurred involving the Streit family. Buck's father had died, and his mother, having raised eight or nine children, decided to really enjoy the rest of her life. Mrs. Streit spent her summers in Paris and her winters in Havana. She spent very little time in Birmingham, but when she did stay there, it was in the deluxe manner. She had wheedled Mr. Streit into building her a beautiful, big home on the crest of the mountain overlooking Birmingham with the idea that they would sell the place. Several times previously he had built large houses which she would furnish from Europe; then they would sell the house "guts, feathers, and all" at a profit. This time though she kept the mansion. Being socially ambitious, Mrs. Streit told Buck and me to invite our best girl friends for dinner at her house, and she would put on a party for us. We wore our tuxedos, the girls wore evening dresses, and we were enjoying a dinner served by several servants. The champagne was some she had brought from Cuba, during Prohibition times, of course. About the time we were finishing our meal, Brice and Marge Streit came in the back door unannounced and in their riding clothes. Brice hollered, "Maw, we came to bottle the homebrew! Do you think it's about ready?" Well, if anybody has ever been deflated, it was Mrs. Streit. There she was serving her guests champagne when her son and daughter-in-law arrived to bottle the homebrew they had made in the basement!

I drove a car at this time and drove back and forth the five miles to school in downtown Birmingham. During World War I, Central High School had burned. Thus I attended high school at first in the temporary school at the former Birmingham Medical College while the replacement to Central High School was being built. When the new school (John Herbert Phillips High School) was completed, I attended it only half a year before going on to the University of Alabama.

During the summer of 1921, I spent a few weeks in Stanford, Kentucky, with Pop's parents, Mr. and Mrs. John Menefee. I remember that I left Birmingham before daylight on July 2 with two men who were friends of Pop's in their big car (a Premier). We arrived in Columbia, Tennessee, that night too late to get supper at the Bethel House Hotel, but the desk clerk in the hotel couldn't believe we had traveled all the way from Birmingham, Alabama, in just one day. It must have been two hundred miles up there! I remember the date because it was the same day Jack Dempsey and Georges Carpentier fought for the world heavyweight championship, and we had stopped along the way a couple of times to see how the fight was progressing.

The next day we went from Columbia to Cave City, Kentucky. The following day (July 4th) the crowd wanting to go through Mammoth Cave was overwhelming, so we got a guide to take us through the cave on the night of July 3rd. We later learned that our guide's name was Floyd Collins. He became famous when he was killed in the bottom of one of Kentucky's caves.

I went on in the car with the two men to Frankfort, then got on an interurban railroad and rode down to Georgetown, Kentucky. From Georgetown I got down to the small town of Stanford, right in the center of the state, some way or other.

Pop's father and mother were both living, and his older brother John Menefee, Jr., was the Probate Judge of that county at the time.

I learned a lot that summer about a lot of things. I didn't know a thing about farming, and the Menefees lived on a horse farm almost in the middle of town. Incidentally, there were a hundred steps going from the town up to their home. Old Man Menefee would sit on the front porch in the evenings; as it began to get dark, he would start shedding his clothes. By dark he was down to his long johns, which he wore even in the summer time, and then he went upstairs and went to bed. He expected me to do the same thing, I imagine. In the mornings just before daylight, he'd wake me up saying, "Jim, it's nearly daylight. It's time to be up. You haven't gotten a thing done today." He was very jovial about it, but he couldn't stand the idea of anybody sleeping after daylight.

During the five or six weeks I spent in Kentucky, I was carried around to visit several places—Boonesboro, Bardstown, Crab Orchard, and Danville. I actually took a trip with John Menefee, Jr., up into one of the "knobs" where we saw people in a place called Ottenheim who were so isolated they had no rural mail carrier come into their town. These people didn't know there had been a world war! They were of German descent, most ingenious, and good farmers, but unbelievably isolated from the world.

There were no laws against children driving automobiles when I was a youth. Anybody big enough to reach the pedals could drive. I must have been about fifteen or sixteen when I made a second trip to Kentucky. This time I drove from Birmingham to Stanford taking Granny, my sister Virginia, and Virginia's good friend Susan Mabry to spend a few days at the Menefee home. I well remember that the only time we had to put the car into low gear was when we'd stop. That was remarkable in those days when cars were not only not very powerful but they were geared so that the driver had to change into a lower gear to go up a steep hill.

The Menefees had a big garden and farm and welcomed visitors with open arms. Just before we arrived, their grandson Sam Menefee, Jr., had visited from New York City. Sam had never seen anything growing except possibly one tree in Brooklyn. One day old man Menefee went out into the garden and brought in some vegetables, and the next day went out into the smoke house and brought in a ham. Sam told him, "I looked all over that garden with you, Grandpa, but I didn't see those hams growing out there anywhere."

Back in Birmingham, near where we lived was a crossroads called Waddell where there was a baseball team which traveled around playing other sandlot teams. Once we went to New Merkle to play. As we were riding in and on a t-model car on our way to New Merkle, we passed by our house. I was riding on the fender or running board because all of us couldn't get in the car at once. As we passed the house, I was smoking a cigarette, and Pop saw me. That night when I got home, he asked me if he hadn't seen me smoking a cigarette that day. I admitted that I had smoked one, and he replied, "Well, you should have let me know that you wanted to smoke. I would have bought you a big black cigar so you could have had a real smoke." I didn't know any better than to say that would be fine. He did buy me a big black cigar, and I got awfully sick smoking it. And I didn't smoke any more for quite a while.

At Waddell where there was also a cow dip. In those days, the health department required that cows be dipped periodically in a trough of antiseptic solution to get rid of tics which caused them to have transmissible diseases; however, the dipping reduced their production of milk. This was a very unpleasant duty as the driver had to drive the cow up to the dipping vat, push it into the vat, and then drive the cow back home. Neither dairy farmers nor owners of one or two cows liked this dipping, but it was required and thus had to be tolerated. On December 14, 1922, I was walking our cow home from having been dipped at Waddell when a man stopped me and gave me the news that my mother had died. Pop and Virginia had gone by train up to Asheville the day before because we knew that Mother was desperately ill, but I heard the news of her death from a man I barely knew.

Mother had had to go back to a sanitarium in Asheville and had been there for about five or six months before she died when I was just fifteen. Her death left our family like a ship without a rudder. My sister and I were still young, my grandmother was getting old, and Pop Menefee was busy traveling trying to make a living for us as a salesman and manager for the Goodyear Company. Granny moved into the house with us, and we continued our lives there for about a year after Mother's death.

After our mother's death, Virginia decided to go to Montevallo to high school, so she and several other girls (Eleanor Willis, Eleanor Moody, Susan Mabry, Emily Reynolds, and Mary Dudley Gray) all went to Montevallo in January 1923 to finish high school. That left Granny and me at home during the week while Pop Menefee was on the road. I didn't have life too rough, but I did have chores to do: transporting the cook back and forth to work, buying groceries, taking clothes to the laundry or dry cleaners, and other little chores which were unusual for a fifteen- year-old boy. For instance, I had to do the banking for the family, getting cash from the bank to buy the necessities and even occasionally depositing a check in the bank. Virginia, Pop, and I were lucky enough to escape tuberculosis at that time; Granny apparently was hyper-immune. Thus we got along pretty well.

Once when Granny and I were visiting Virginia in Montevallo on a Sunday afternoon, I was stopped for speeding. I had been up at the college and was headed toward the middle of the "big city" of Montevallo down a very rough unpaved road at about twenty miles per hour when a man stepped out in front of me. He hailed me down and asked me how fast I was going. When I told him that I had been going about twenty miles per hour, he said, "That's exactly what I thought; the speed limit is fifteen." He hauled me before the local judge or justice of the peace, and they extracted five dollars of my scant funds before they let me go on about my business. Believe me, there have been many times when I have since flown over the city of Montevallo and paid my respects to them by use of the relief tube which was in the airplane, but I have never again visited the town nor do I intend to do so. I might have to spend a nickel in that town!

Pop Menefee was a prince! No man could have been better to a boy than he was to me, and he was equally as good to my sister. He was thoughtful, considerate, kind, and anything good you could think of.

I was so anxious to become independent and earn my own livelihood that I worked hard as a student. I rarely missed a day of school. I was a hard student, not an excellent one, and through this hard work was able earn enough credits to go off to college when I was still fifteen.

A little while after Virginia had left home, my grandmother got a job as maitre d' or major-domo of a hotel restaurant in Birmingham. She was the chief buyer and supervisor, as well as maitre d' of this hotel, and in addition to a small salary was furnished food and a place to live in the Ridgeway Apartments for herself and Virginia. Not long afterwards I went off to college, and Pop moved into a hotel. Thus we gave up the house and broke up housekeeping.

3

Alabama and Girls

WHEN I WENT TO COLLEGE IN THE SUMMER OF 1923, I had as a trunk in which I put my books and clothes an old sample trunk which had been Pop Menefee's. That summer, I was admitted as a conditional student because I hadn't actually finished high school, and I took political science and English. Though I began my college days early (a couple of months before my sixteenth birthday), I was not the youngest student at all; there was one student, William Inge Hill, who was twelve years old.

We had a state law in Alabama at that time that anyone who was twenty-one years old and wanted to attend the University of Alabama could do so. But even then there were only a limited number of boys and girls who had attended high school and wanted to attend the university. We had only sixteen hundred students—no sixteen hundred boys and girls—attending school at the University but only about five or six students, certainly not many more than that. It wasn't all that great a thing to go to a university at that time. (And there was only one university in Alabama at the time, the University of Alabama at Tuscaloosa. There was a Polytechnic Institute at Auburn, and there were colleges at Montevallo, Howard, Birmingham-Southern, and elsewhere, but there was only one university in the state.)

As a first year pre-medical student I had a full schedule. I studied English, math, chemistry, biology, German, and military training. It was about all a fellow could handle at one time. There were perhaps fifty in our beginning pre-med class. There were boys there who had no idea that they wanted to be doctors, and they soon decided or had it decided for them that they weren't going to be pre-med students. They became law or engineering or literary students or something else, but they couldn't stand the pressure of having quite so many classes. I would love to have been able to study astronomy and psychology, but there was no place on my schedule for such courses. I was only a B+ student; had I been an A+ student, I might have been able to add psychology and astronomy to my curriculum, but I certainly was not that.

During my second year at the University, I was invited to join a group called Kappa Psi, a medical fraternity composed of pre-medical and medical students. I had not been invited to join a social fraternity, that is a national one. I had been invited to join a local social fraternity, but I was not equipped either socially or financially to join one of those which were more socially desirable. Kappa Psi was one of three or four medical fraternities at Alabama at the time; it, like the others, was more or less an eating society. After all, freshman medical students smelled so bad (from their hours in the anatomy lab) that they couldn't hope to eat in a boarding house and thus of necessity belonged to a medical fraternity to have a place to eat.

Our group was by no means an affluent one. Only one student at the University had a car, and there were no married students then. We had boys in medicine trying to eke out a living by waiting on tables, but they didn't do very well because the courses in anatomy and pathology were so rigorous that they required about half of a student's waking hours to pass.

During my sophomore year, my grades fell very rapidly. I had become engrossed in a female student, and while I was busy courting this girl, I didn't have time to study. One day I received a letter from my stepfather telling me to meet him in his office on Saturday morning at 9 o'clock; he wanted to see me. I immediately knew that I was going to get a raking over the coals and went prepared for that, but I didn't know exactly what I was going to hear. When I arrived, my most understanding stepfather told me, "Jim, your grades have fallen from good to fair (a much worse grade), and I know that you've either been chasing some girl, drinking too much whiskey, or not studying enough, and probably a combination of those things."

Well, I hadn't been drinking, but I had been chasing this gal pretty hard, and consequently I hadn't been studying enough.

Pop then further reminded me, "There isn't anything that the professors are trying to teach you that you already know. Certainly you've got to study more and chase women less or you'll flunk out of school or at least not get into medical school. You just must attend to your business better."

Well, I understood that and subsequently did do better. In fact, in the second half of my sophomore year, I had pulled my grades up so that I was one of the few who went out under an oak tree with one of our professors and formed an honorary society of pre-med students which is now a national institution called Alpha Epsilon Delta. I take great pride in being one of the founders of that organization after having had a good talk with my stepfather.

The idea of running around the country in an automobile was unusual to say the least. But one Saturday, Buck Streit called me and

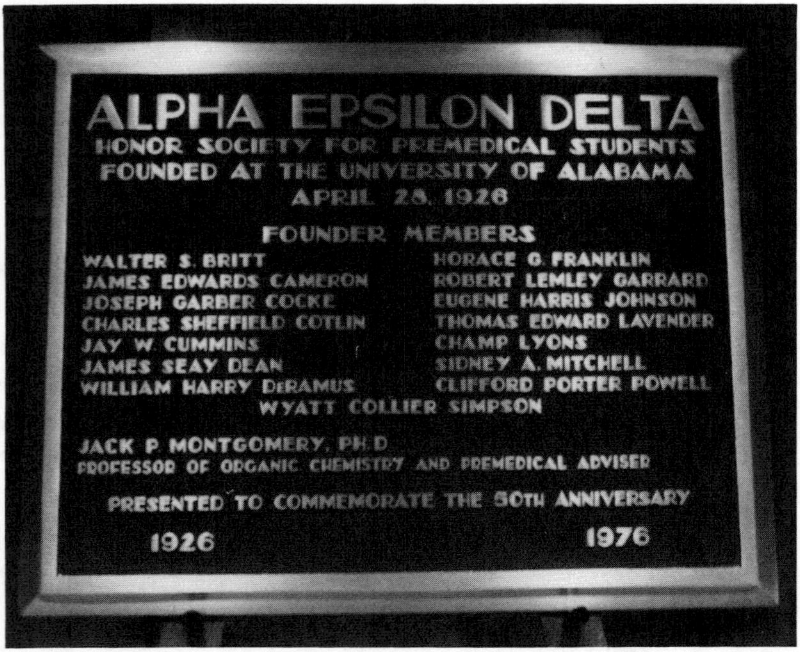

Plaque commemorating Alpha Epsilon Delta, premedical honor society—University of Alabama.

suggested that we go to Memphis to have a good time. A girl whom I had been dating at the University lived across the river from Memphis, so I agreed that the thing for us to do was go to Memphis that night. We both worked all day, and after supper we struck out to go to Memphis. We had passed Walker County and were somewhere in the western part of Alabama when we both went to sleep. We waked up off the road and in a corn field. We had run off the road but luckily had not hit a tree or anything. All we had to do was back the car up and get back on the road. We went on to Memphis, but we didn't have nearly as good a time as we had thought we would have. Furthermore, we came back home dead tired after a weekend of traveling.

Another incident which happened during my years at Alabama involved a very proper young English instructor named Brooks Forehand. Forehand lived, as I did, in old Clark Hall which was part library and part rooming house, and one night several of us were having a party and very probably got too loud. Anyway, after a while we heard a knocking on our door and a male voice warning us to quiet down. Someone went to the door but instead of opening it called out, "Who's there?"

The voice answered, "It's me, Brooks Forehand!"

The quick-witted fellow on the inside replied, "Ah, go on whoever you are. If you were Brooks Forehand, you would have said, 'It's I, not it's me."

Well, we later learned that it was Brooks Forehand, but he was so embarrassed at having made this grammatical mistake that he sheepishly returned to his room and tolerated our loudness for the rest of the evening.

4

Medical School: 'Enough Anatomy to Pick a Chicken'

IN THOSE DAYS, PRE-MEDICAL STUDY CONSISTED OF three years of undergraduate study. Then with good enough grades and completion of certain required courses, a student could be admitted to medical school without having an undergraduate degree. He might, of course, choose to go a fourth year and complete a degree, but that was not a requirement. Thus after three years, I gained admittance to the University of Alabama's medical school (without a high school diploma or an undergraduate degree).

In the first and second years of medical school (which was all the University of Alabama offered at the time), we had good and bad professors. The good professors were rare; we had a bunch of mediocre hacks for the most part, but we had one outstanding man named George T. Pack.

Dr. Pack was a brain and a fabulous person, and I take great pride in having been a student in his class. Pack was rather young. At the age of twenty-seven or twenty-eight, he was a full professor and worked in some Birmingham hospitals as their pathologist on the weekends, commuting on the local train between Birmingham and Tuscaloosa. Dr. Pack worked from 6:00 a.m. until midnight every day. He finally became one of the great doctors of the world, the author of a textbook on cancer, and the editor of a series of medical texts, as well as teaching at Columbia,

Harvard, and Yale at the same time after he had left the University of Alabama.

In addition to teaching us pathology, Dr. Pack also taught minor surgery and was the assistant dean of the medical school. One day he announced that he had a book which he would award as a prize to the student in the class who learned knot-tying to the greatest proficiency. In other words, we had to learn to tie knots three or four different ways. The book was a beautiful monograph, and I was very anxious to win it. Thus I worked very hard learning knot-tying. Then on the last day before the contest, Dr. Pack announced that every student in the class had to participate in the contest. My good friend Jim Farrior had not been interested in knot-tying at all, so he got me to show him how to tie the various knots on the night before the contest. When he went up the next day and beat me and won the book, I was greatly disillusioned because my student had beaten me.

Another thing I remember about the course in minor surgery was that we had to learn intubation. In those days many people had diphtheria. One of the ways of keeping the patient with diphtheria alive was to put a metal tube down through the larynx into the trachea. This procedure was called intubation. I had skipped the class when that procedure was being demonstrated, and Dr. Pack was aware that I had missed that class. When the time came for a practical examination in minor surgery, each student who had missed a class was given the assignment of doing the task which had been taught in the class he had missed. I got the task of intubing a live goat. Now a goat has a long face, and to put an intubation tube down a goat must be at least three times as hard as putting one down a human. Still Dr. Pack was five-star teacher and a real brain, and I never enjoyed anything more than having him for a teacher.

I can remember another incident which will furnish further some idea of what kind of brain Dr. Pack was. About that time Sinclair Lewis's novel, *Arrowsmith*, about a medical student, was published. I had bought a copy of Arrowsmith and had put it in the windowsill while I worked on pathologic specimens one afternoon. When Dr. Pack came along and saw the book, he said, "I haven't read that book yet. Do you mind if I borrow it to read this afternoon?" Of course, I told him he could borrow it, so he took the book to his laboratory and brought it back in about an hour telling me that he had thoroughly enjoyed reading it. I just knew he was a damn showoff and couldn't possibly have read it in that short time, but the man had a photographic mind. Months later, I asked him if he remembered the scene in Arrowsmith where the fat boy had gone to take an examination. He replied, "Oh, sure, I remember that; it's on page 316. He ran his pencil down the rail fence to make a noise like he was walking through a graveyard." And that's exactly where that scene was — on page 316 — and Dr. Pack remembered everything about it.

About that time also I was enamored of a girl in Birmingham named Selinda Taylor. Her father was an eminent surgeon, Dr. Adrian Taylor. Dr. Taylor had spent twenty years as Professor of Surgery at Peking Union Medical School, the foremost American medical institution in the Orient. When he returned to the United States, he had gone through Harvard Medical School; thus he had two medical degrees, the only man I ever knew who had such qualifications. There were other outstanding doctors in Birmingham at the time, but Dr. Taylor was by far the greatest of all. He did brain surgery, thoracic surgery, gynecologic surgery, hemorrhoidal surgery, vascular surgery, and any other kind of surgery. He was an all-around surgeon. One day Dr. Pack asked me if I wasn't dating Selinda Taylor. When I told him that I was, he replied, "Well, I know her father very well. I often examine specimens for him when I'm working in Birmingham. But I tell you, I believe I'd rather have the fellow for my surgeon than for a father-in-law." So he put me on the right track at that time.

Incidentally, Dr. Pack was called on more than once to treat some of the crowned heads of Europe and South America. He and Dr. J. Marion Sims were the two doctors from Alabama who were ever so honored.

One teacher who stands out in my mind was a fellow named John Shining, a Russian immigrant who had come to this country after the Russian Revolution. As he went through Ellis Island, his long Russian name had been changed to John Shining. He had painted signs on buildings in New York for a few years before coming to Alabama to work as an instructor in the department of anatomy. The amazing thing about John was that if a student gave him a perfect recitation, he wrote down in his grade book a 70. That was the highest grade he gave anybody; seventy was also the minimum passing grade in the medical school. If he asked you how many fingers and toes you had and you told him you had eight fingers, two thumbs, two big toes, and eight smaller toes for a total of twenty, he wrote down a seventy.

If a student questioned the grade, he justified it by saying, "Well, the man who wrote the book on anatomy doesn't know everything; certainly I couldn't give him 100 percent. The professor doesn't know as much as the man who wrote the book; I couldn't give him 90 percent. I don't know as much as the professor; I couldn't give myself an 80 percent grade. You are just a student, so I'll give you a 70 percent grade." And that's the way it went.

Paul Lyle White

One of my fellow students in the first year of medical school was from Cherokee County. His name was Paul Lyle White. He wasn't the Paul Dudley White from Boston, and he made it very clear that there was a distinction. Paul was quite a character. He devoted a good deal of his time to liquor drinking and would go into ventricular fibrillation when he would drink too much. When he realized that his heart was racing too fast, he would devoutly swear that he would never take another drink. About that time his heart would slow down spontaneously, and he'd say, "Jim, don't you reckon I'd better have another drink to kinda help my nerves?"

Paul lived in the medical fraternity house where study was the main ingredient. The house rules were lax, but we tried to keep the place where we could study there. One of the rules of the house was that women of questionable character were not to be admitted. Well, Paul brought in a girl one night and they spent the night there. At the next meeting of the house committee, someone suggested that Paul was subject to being fined for having brought such a woman into the house. But Paul said, "Now, wait just a G-- d--- minute! I want you to understand that there wasn't any question about that girl's character at all!" And according to the wording of the rule, we couldn't fine Paul for having brought in a girl of questionable character.

On another occasion Paul was being raked over the coals about something. He became a little recalcitrant and said that he wanted to let us know that he wasn't under "any obli-God-damn-gation" to anybody in that organization.

Paul didn't devote much time to study, but he wore a pair of glasses on a string, and with the glasses hung over his nose he looked very studious and thought he was impressing the professors, particularly in anatomy class. However, he wasn't. When the final examination time came in anatomy class, Dr. Noah saw Paul come into the room and said, "Mr. White, you can't take the final examination."

"Well, Dr. Noah, why can't I?" Paul asked.

Dr. Noah replied, "Mr. White, you don't know enough anatomy to pick a chicken! You might pass anatomy, and if you did, you might get to be a doctor, and that would be a sin against the whole of creation!"

So Paul packed his bags, and when the rest of us got home from the examination, Paul had gone back to Cherokee County. He later became a chiropractor, and though I'm sure he's long dead, we know some people from his home town who also remember him as being quite a character.

Group Two

During my second year in medical school, we were divided into groups of four students. I was a member of what was known as Group Two. In addition to myself, the group consisted of Boyd "Boy Dog" Burkehart, Jim "Blue" Farrior, and Carmel "Hog" Roberts. These friends were quite a group of characters.

Burkehart had attended several other universities, including Indiana and Arizona, before he arrived at Alabama. During his first semester as a medical student, his father had agreed to pay only for his tuition and books. His mother sent him one dollar and a carton of cigarettes per week. So he had to depend on his friends for food and lodging until he could prove to his father that he would make passing grades. Yet Boyd was so affable that everyone liked him immediately; through the generosity of his girl friend he was even able to attend all the out-of-town football games that season.

I had met Jim Farrior during my first summer at Alabama when we had lived in the same rooming house. He had quite a way with the women which earned him the nickname of "Bluebeard" which we shortened to "Blue."

"Hog," a name he preferred over his real name of Carmel, was the son of a doctor in Dothan. He was nice looking, most affable, and more of a politician than a student. He finally became president of the Florida Medical Association.

That crazy Burkehart was always making some reference to the great achievements of Group Two. Burkehart's wide experience in college attendance had at least taught him to give the appearance of being a great student. He was an accomplished pseudo-student at least. Farrior was a good student; Hog Roberts was a poor student and I was a mediocre one, so we had all gradations in Group Two. After two years of medical school, we broke up and all went to separate schools to finish our medical degrees. Roberts went to the University of Arkansas; Farrior went to Northwestern University in Chicago; I went to Tulane; and Burkehart went to the University of Indiana. Thus we didn't see each other for many years, but during that year the association of Group Two was wonderful.

Altogether, my second year in medical school was devoted largely to study and very little else. Had it not been for the contacts I had with the hilarious people such as the members of Group Two, the year would have been a complete washout. I accomplished nothing, but I did get to meet and know some very interesting people.

Doctors

During these years there were several doctors in Birmingham, in addition to Dr. Adrian Taylor, whom I remember well.

One was Cecil Gaston, a procto-enterologist. That meant that he specialized in treating hemorrhoids. Gaston was a very nice gentleman, and he was widely known for the large fees which he charged. However, he devoted two mornings a week to treatment of patients in the charity wards at Hillman Hospital. If any of his regular patients gave him any trouble about the enormous fees he charged them, he would tell them they could have come down to Hillman Hospital and been operated on there free.

Another doctor I remember well was Marie Dabney, a urologist and gynecologist. He was also a nice gentleman and good doctor.

In contrast, another prominent doctor was the sorriest of all those I knew. He had a big following among his fellow Catholics. I later learned that many people follow their religion when choosing their doctors. Incidentally, he was the father-in-law of one of Birmingham's early brain surgeons, Garber Galbraith. Galbraith was a well-trained, good neurosurgeon, but his father-in-law should have been chopping cotton. He had no business working on sick people at all.

Another popular doctor was Earl Drennen, a society doctor who was a favorite among the bridge-playing, diamond-wearing women of the city. He was more popular than capable.

Summers

During the summer of 1924, after my freshman year, I worked at whatever jobs I could find around Birmingham, but I can't remember where I lived. I do remember that after my second year I worked in the lab washing bottles and doing other menial jobs at what is now Lloyd Noland Hospital, then T. C. I. hospital. This experience was most valuable to me because I learned some laboratory techniques. I learned more what to do than why it was done or what the results would be, but gradually it was thrust upon me that I learned some of the art of medicine in a reverse manner. You can't imagine someone learning to do a Widal test (for typhoid fever) or Wassermann (for syphilis) before he knew what he was testing for, but that's the way it occurred in my case.

My work at the hospital provided me with board, room, and laundry; that was all I was paid that first summer I worked there. The next summer I again worked at T. C. I. Hospital, but then I earned board, room, laundry, and twenty-five dollars per month. The third summer I got fifty dollars per month, and in the fourth summer my salary went up to seventy-five dollars while interns there earned only fifty dollars. Thus when I went back there as an intern after finishing medical school, I took a reduction in salary. However, these small amounts were not inconsiderable to a boy who wanted to learn medicine, and fifty dollars per month was more than many interns were paid in many elegant hospitals around the world.

5

Tulane: Hard Work and Good Friends

THEN IN THE FALL OF 1928 I WENT TO TULANE, AND there a whole new world opened up. I lived at 2006 Canal Street with James Porter (Shim) Collier and Bob Cochran, both of Tuscaloosa, who were seniors when I was a junior. Those were our clinical years when we saw patients in Charity Hospital, which was a completely different experience from the didactic courses we had taken before.

One friend who went through premed and medical school (both at Alabama and Tulane) with me was Red Williams from Hartford, Alabama. Red, Lester Crowell, and I shared an apartment in New Orleans during my second year there. While Lester and I studied enough to get by pretty well, Red was out courting the girls about half that time. He was not bad about drinking, but he would come home late at night, raise the windows to let in the cold air, and make lots of noise. That didn't set well with either Lester or me, so one night we decided to get even with him. We took a wine bottle, filled it with chips of ice, tied a string around the cork, and tied the other end of the string to the foot of Red's bed. That night when Red came home about midnight and climbed into bed, he immediately felt the cold bottle of ice in his bed; when he jumped up and pulled the bottle out from under the covers, he pulled out the cork, spreading the ice and water all up and down his bed.

He wasn't very happy about our prank, but he got our message and from then on was much quieter when he came in after his dates.

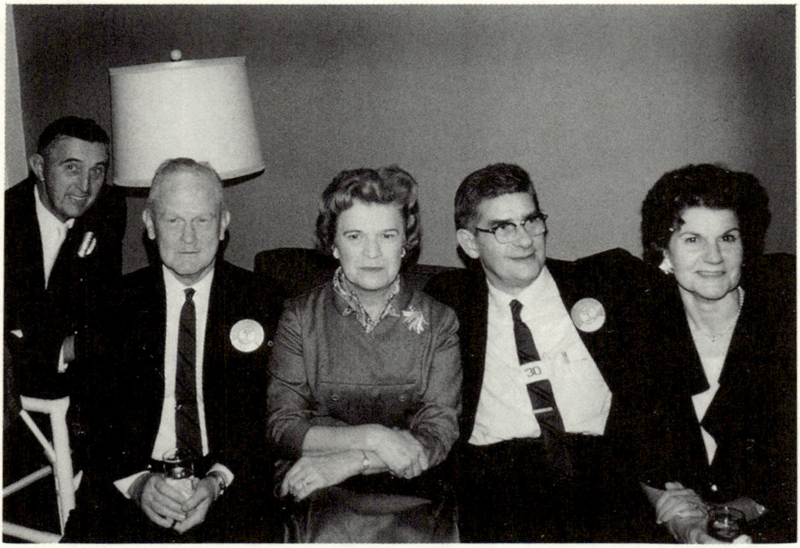

Tulane roommates and their wives: Jim Cameron, Frazier "Red" Williams, Edith Cameron, Lester Crowell, and Elaine Crowell—at a reunion in 1965.

When Red finished Tulane, he specialized in treatment of ears, nose, and throat and set up his practice on the edge of Washington, D.C. The only times I saw Red after our school years were when we would attend class reunions or visit my sister Virginia in Falls Church, Virginia.

My other roommate, Lester Crowell, was from the little town of Lincolnton, North Carolina. Lester had had polio when he was nine months old and could get around only with the aid of a crutch, a cane, and a brace on one leg. In those days before elevators were commonplace, some of the buildings in which we had classes were three storied. When Lester had a class on the second or third story of such a building, Johnny Menville and I would form a chair with our arms and carry Lester up the stairs. We also carried him to football games or dances when they were not accessible to the handicapped. And Lester did enjoy going to dances. He'd get all dressed up in his tuxedo and have as much fun as anybody. As he liked to say, "I may not be able to dance, but I can intermission as well as anybody."

Lester's father once made a trip to New Orleans to see how his son was getting along. On this trip he took me aside and asked for my help.

Lester, using crutches as he did, quickly wore out the armpits of his coats, yet he was indifferent about the matter or too tight with his money to care about clothes. So Dr. Crowell asked me to go downtown and buy Lester two suits and send the bill to him. And he added that when those wore out, I was to go back and buy two more. Dr. Crowell Sr. was a surgeon and had his own hospital in Lincolnton. Later Lester served as an internist there, and his brother became the administrator or manager of this hospital. After he finished medical school, Lester married, became the father of five children, and practiced medicine actively for fifty years. In fact, I was quite flattered that he named his only son, Gordon Cameron Crowell, for me.

When we were seniors, we actually delivered some babies for some of the people who were in the lower echelon of the New Orleans social world. The black bag of the doctor furnished us protection against thugs and thieves, so we could get to the place where a woman was about to deliver a baby. If we ran into complications, we were allowed to call for help. In such cases, an ambulance came to pick the woman up and carry her to Charity Hospital, so actually we were the equivalent of midwives. I suppose we delivered about ten babies apiece as midwives. We also attended complicated deliveries of ten to twenty more babies during our junior and senior years. Those were all done at the hospital under the supervision of the Professor of Gynecology and Obstetrics; this experience was quite enlightening.

One of my friends at Tulane who was also a professor was named Dr. Ruttock; he was quite an adept obstetrician and taught me a good deal. Another professor of obstetrics was Dr. King, an uncle of my senior roommate, Frazier "Red" Williams. Dr. King was quite helpful to us in some ways.

We had many other professors and many courses. Believe me, during the last two years of medicine the students studied so many things it is impossible to enumerate all of them. They included psychiatry, tropical medicine, dermatology, urology, obstetrics, surgery, pediatrics, and others—about seventeen subjects which we studied at the same time. And for the most part, each professor thought his was the only subject we were studying.

One day I ran into a young fellow whom I didn't know. He began giving me a hard time about not keeping up with my work on the wards,

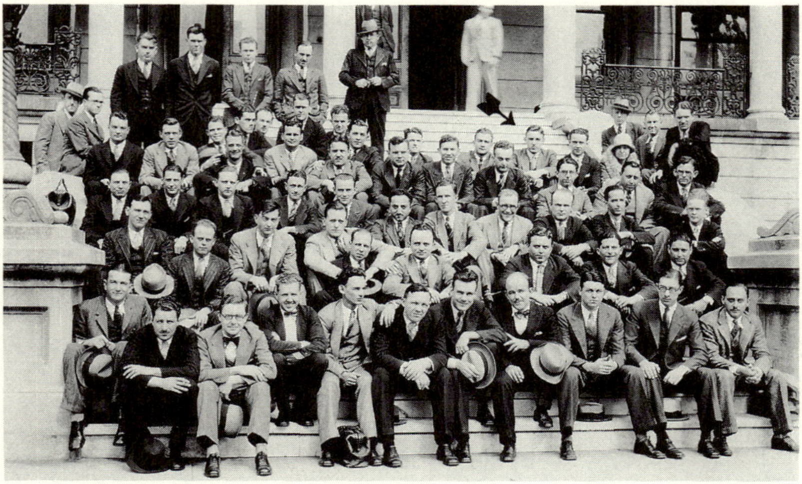

Tulane Medical School Class of 1930 (Jim Cameron fifth row back, third person from right seated on steps).

but I assured him that I was working as hard as I could work and that we had a good many other courses we were taking at the same time and I just couldn't give any more time to that job. Later I learned that he was the new Professor of Surgery and I had made a faux pas.

Among my dearest friends while I was in school in New Orleans were Johnny Menville and Warren Herbert, both local boys whose fathers were on the medical school faculty at Tulane. Johnny Menville's father was a professor of radiology, and Warren Herbert's father was an assistant professor in the Department of Obstetrics. But in spite of these entrees at Tulane, medical school was a grind.

While I was a student in Charity Hospital in New Orleans, a small group of students was being lectured to by one of the instructors in pediatrics. A new patient was admitted to the large ward, and the teacher delegated one student to go see what was ailing this new patient. The student was gone only a couple of minutes and returned with a diagnosis of measles. The professor asked how he knew that was the correct diagnosis: was the child broken out or did he have Koplick spots? Without any hesitation, the student replied, "Oh, I know he has the measles; his grandmother says he has."

6

'I Knew That Young Puppy Would Come to No Good'

WHEN I GRADUATED FROM TULANE ON JUNE 11, 1930, I went to work as an intern at the Employees' Hospital of the Tennessee Coal, Iron, and Railroad Co., otherwise known as T. C. I. Hospital. Interns at some hospitals were given room, board, and laundry but paid nothing at all. They only had to work about 160 hours a week with an hour or two off to go to the barber shop and a few hours otherwise. There have been times during internships when the boys were on duty twenty-four hours a day for a month at a time with one hour off to go to the barber shop. Now they didn't actually work all that time; they worked only about twelve hours a day, but the rest of the time they were on call. They had to stay right in the hospital and were subject to being called all during the hours between midnight and dawn. Sometimes there was a long stint when they went unrelieved, but that was expected. It was nothing unusual in those days for a doctor to want to work where there was lots to be done and lots to be learned and there was no other way to teach it than by precept and example.

The next echelon was the resident who worked nearly as much as the intern did. On up the ladder of medicine, doctors worked a little less, but they still thought nothing of working about seventy-five hours per week.

At many hospitals interns did laboratory work because technicians were not available to do this work. We were fortunate at T. C. I. to have a well-trained corps of people to do lab work, so interns were spared that duty. Interns were allowed to do anything they were capable of doing and were trained to do. Internship was just a continuation of medical school; that's the way it was thought of by Dr. Lloyd Noland and thus the way it was. We got to participate in surgery first as second assistant, then as assistant, and after we had been assisting at surgery for several months, we were allowed to do very simple cases with the boss serving on the other side of the table as assistant. For instance, I got to do a few appendectomies and a few hernia operations with Dr. Noland assisting me, and this experience was a tremendous help to me. In many hospitals, interns did not get enough training in surgery to be allowed to do operations themselves, no matter with how much assistance.

One amusing thing which happened during my internship involved my Uncle Andy. A Miss Roland was the night supervisor in the hospital. Miss Roland was middle aged and not pretty by any means. She also had a bad habit of coming around to the room where the intern on emergency call was sleeping to ask sometimes trivial questions. One night when I was on call, she had been around two or three times to ask me different questions. Then the switchboard operator called to ask if Miss Roland was there in my room. I told her "No." Just a few minutes later, the operator called again asking the same question. The third time she called, not more than half an hour later, I answered, "Yes, but we're in bed together and don't want to be disturbed."

The young woman who was the operator thought my answer was hilariously funny, especially since just about that time Miss Roland walked up to her desk. The operator then told Miss Roland what I had said. Miss Roland, having no sense of humor, was incensed that anybody had impinged upon her reputation.

A few days later it happened that Uncle Andy was admitted to the hospital to be treated for acute alcoholism. That night when Miss Roland was being briefed by the day nurses on new patients and was informed that Dr. Cameron had been admitted for acute alcoholism, she (thinking of me) said, "Yes, I knew that young puppy would come to no good at all!"

Recently we have had the widely publicized trial in Los Angeles in which O. J. Simpson was accused of killing his ex-wife and a male friend of hers. Domestic trouble always reminds me of something which happened when I was an intern. We had a woman brought to the hospital one night whose husband had hit her over the head with meat platter. It had parted her scalp, and she was bleeding profusely. We sewed up her scalp and kept her in the hospital overnight so we could x ray her the next morning to be sure she didn't have a skull fracture.

The next morning, we determined that her skull was not fractured, and the wound looked all right, so we told her she could go home. But in filling out the papers, we were required to state where she was going. I asked her if she were going back home to that man who had hit her over the head with the meat platter.

"Oh, yeah," she replied, "he's been good to me this year. Las' year he broke my laig."

I was never sick a day while I was in college. When I went to medical school in New Orleans, I was associated with people who had tuberculosis. The disease was very common in New Orleans. My first inkling of any trouble was on a routine tuberculin test which all students had to take. I had a strong reaction showing that at some time or other I had come in contact with the tubercle bacillus. That was all it showed; I didn't have tuberculosis then but had been exposed to it.

All during my college years, I had really not had any home. I spent nine months per year in school in Tuscaloosa or New Orleans and the other three months of each year at Fairfield at T. C. I. Hospital. During my last year in Tuscaloosa, Pop Menefee had married a widow, Buford Henderson. They and her daughter, Nettie Henderson, lived in Birmingham, and they visited me in Tuscaloosa occasionally and were very kind to me, but I did not consider their home my home.

In 1930 my sister married Emmett Girard "Todd" Craig, an engineer who had been sent to Alabama to oversee the building of Martin Dam for the parent company of Alabama Power Company. Todd and Virginia lived in Birmingham only a very short while before he was transferred to New York.

7

Asheville and Highland Baptist

IN 1931, ONLY A FEW WEEKS BEFORE I FINISHED MY internship at T. C. I. Hospital, I was diagnosed with tuberculosis. I didn't know what to do. My father was called on to help me, but he didn't respond very well. Dr. Noland loaned me fifty dollars a month for nine months, and Granny gave me twenty-five dollars per month to eke out my treatment in a sanitarium in Asheville, North Carolina.

In Asheville I lay in bed for those nine months of 1931 and 1932, allowed to get up to bathe only once a week and to sit at a table to eat my meals. Otherwise, I had to lie in bed. There I was allowed to read, and with no radio or television, I did read a great deal. I read a good deal of medical literature including one extensive work on chest x rays. I read *The Decline and Fall of the Roman Empire* in twelve volumes, *The Outline of History*, and the Bible from cover to cover. I just called words; I didn't read any of these works thoroughly or understandingly, but I did attempt to read them. I also read many other things while I was there.

When I got out of the hospital in Asheville, I was completely at loose ends. A Dr. Huffines, a urologist in Asheville, took me into his office as an assistant at five dollars per day. I worked there for several months until Dr. Huffines decided he couldn't afford to pay me so much, and I returned to Birmingham. Meanwhile, with all this money I had been earning, I had bought a car. It was six years old and barely movable, but that's what I returned to Birmingham in. I had a room at the Menefee house until I got a job as a resident at the Highland Baptist Hospital.

Then I was all set up with board, room, laundry, and seventy-five dollars per month. At Highland Baptist I earned a base salary of fifty dollars and operated the pharmacy to earn the extra twenty-five dollars per month. This meant I had to dish out all medicines and make up the solutions that were given intravenously, such as glucose. I also ran the laboratory. I was doing all right except that we didn't have enough patients to justify two residents, Tom Wolford and me, and Tom Wolford outranked me. Although there were some very excellent surgeons there, I wasn't learning much and didn't have enough work to entertain me, to say the least.

It was not the best of times in 1932. The small hospital in which I worked actually had a boarder who found that he could rent a room in a hospital cheaper than he could live in a hotel. So he kept his belongings in the hospital while he left on Mondays and went out to sell burial supplies to various undertakers around the country. On weekends he returned to the hospital. As a divorcee he found that living in the hospital was nice because there were lots of young nurses around. The hospital management also saw an advantage in this arrangement since there were many empty rooms in the hospital and no chance of their being filled.

There was also a doctor who was a patient in the hospital at that time. He had been in for a hemorrhoidectomy and being heavily insured stayed in the hospital all during the winter of 1931–32. Of course, by football season of 1932 he had recovered sufficiently that he and his pretty young nurse left the hospital to watch football games sitting on the hard bleachers and have a drink or two of whiskey, but after each game they would return to the hospital.

One of the outstanding doctors practicing at Highland Baptist at the time was the very eminent internist, Dr. Seale Harris, who was widely-known as the doctor who first described hyper-insulinism which was known for a long time as Harris's disease. Dr. Harris introduced me to Dr. T., a patient in the hospital. Dr. T., from Meridian, Mississippi, had practiced medicine for many years then had become an embalmer and funeral director. A long-time patient of Dr. Harris, he was known to have peptic ulcer disease. Of late he had been vomiting most of what he ate and losing weight rapidly. Dr. Harris had me record his history in detail, examine him thoroughly, and record my findings for his chart. We had no interns, so we residents did such scut work.

After Dr. Harris studied the x ray, he determined that the patient had an almost complete obstruction of the pylorus (the junction of the stomach and small intestine).

Then Dr. Harris called in his good friend, Dr. Lee Turlington, a good doctor and nice gentleman, but one who had limited his practice to gynecology. He persuaded the gynecologist that his patient needed surgery, but the outstanding surgeon of Birmingham was out of town. Besides, the gynecologist had at times assisted at gastric surgery during his early training (about fifteen years before).

The gynecologist-turned-gastric-surgeon did a beautiful gastroenterostomy on the undertaker while the internist looked over his shoulder, and relief and recovery came rapidly. The man's stomach healed well; physician-turned-undertaker returned to Mississippi in a couple of weeks; and the gynecologist-turned-gastric-surgeon lived on for many years. He later became president of the Southern Medical Association, the second-largest medical association in America. Many years later, I had him do a gynecological procedure on my wife because I never forgot that if a piece of intestine were accidentally cut, he was perfectly capable of doing intestinal surgery too!

In contrast to these excellent doctors, we had one doctor in that hospital who was completely incapable of operating on anyone, but because times were hard and he did keep some of the beds filled, he was allowed to operate there. One day I had the duty of helping him do a gall bladder operation. When he had about finished with the gall bladder operation, he was ready to turn the patient over and do a hemorrhoidectomy on her, and then he said he'd see if he could do a vaginal repair at the same time. In much disgust I left the operating room; he had been about two hours in doing the first surgery and had done it poorly, and I was not interested in further mutilation of that patient. I don't think he proceeded with the hemorrhoidectomy.

There were other things which went on at that hospital which are hard to believe. For instance, I was robbed while there. After being paid seventy-five dollars in cash one payday, I put the money in my top bureau drawer and went to eat lunch. When I returned, I found that my money was gone. As it happened, the hospital telephone operator's office was right across the hall from my first floor room. She told me that my friend had gone into my room while I had been gone; however, when she described the "friend," he turned out to be a traveling salesman whom I didn't know but whom I had seen once and had noticed that he had two thumbs on one hand. I told the Birmingham police that I had been robbed almost certainly by a man with two thumbs on his right hand, yet they still never found him or my money. Thus from then on I had little faith in the Birmingham police department.

About Christmas time of 1932, Dr. Seale Harris came to me and told me he knew that because the hospital had so few patients I was not getting much out of my residency there. He suggested that perhaps I would like to go to Eclectic, Alabama, where the town's one doctor had been shot by the pharmacist and was not expected to recover. Some of the people of Eclectic had been Dr. Harris's patients and had appealed to him for help in locating a new doctor. He said that there were fine people down in Elmore County, many of whom he knew well. Furthermore, this was a good farming community where the people were all eating regularly (which was not true at the time in Birmingham). Thus, I with my missionary soul and being more or less a social outcast with no home and still single in those days, had only to worry about how I was going to repay those debts I had accumulated to finish medical school and to recuperate from tuberculosis. All together I owed about thirty-five hundred dollars, and that was pressing on my mind when I was only making seventy-five dollars per month at the hospital.

I told Pop about the possibility of my going to Eclectic. He agreed that I was just marking time at Highland Baptist Hospital and encouraged me by saying that if I wanted to try private practice, this seemed to be the time to do so. On a cold and rainy day in late December 1932, he and I drove to Eclectic in his Goodyear Company car to look over the situation.

After I talked to a few people there, I told them I had decided I would come there to practice. I came back to Birmingham, but a few days later developed the flu; while I was in bed in the hospital for two or three days, some people of Eclectic telephoned to know if I were still coming. I assured them that I was as soon as I was able. So on the last day of 1932 I packed all my worldly possessions, including about seventy-five dollars worth of most essential instruments which I had bought, in the back of my little worn-out coupe and moved to Eclectic, Alabama, to begin the real practice of medicine.

8

Thanks to Dr. Owsley

DURING THE WINTER OF 1933, I LIVED IN THE HOtel in Eclectic, in a corner room with a telephone and a lavatory in the room. I got three good square meals per day and had a room by myself with a fireplace which I never lighted. For this I paid only twenty-five dollars per month. The outhouse was about one hundred yards from the hotel, and the barber shop where I went to take a bath was just across the street.

After I had lived in Eclectic for about a year, a Mr. Fant, the vocational agriculture teacher, became the County Agent for Chilton County. He moved to Clanton and rented his house, including the chickens in the yard, to me for the sum of fifteen dollars per month. In January 1934, Granny and I moved into Mr. Fant's house, which had indoor plumbing and running water, one of the few houses in Eclectic with such luxuries.

My office was in the back of a drugstore. There I had to prepare any kind of intravenous solutions in my own small laboratory. This job involved distilling the water, then adding salt or glucose to make saline or glucose solutions. I also had to make up Unna's paste for the treatment of varicose ulcers. And though I didn't make up the plaster of Paris, I did wrap bandages with plaster of Paris to treat broken bones. So the treatment was primitive, but it was better than the people had had available up to that time.

I am reminded that we had only primitive medicines then, and there were only a few medicines which were really efficacious. Morphine was effective for the relief of pain; ether or chloroform could be given as an anesthetic; quinine was effective in the treatment of malaria. Salvarsan or neo-salvarsan was partially effective when used with mercury and bismuth in the treatment of syphilis. Digitalis was a great help in the treatment of certain types of heart disease. There were one or two mercurial diuretics which were somewhat, though not greatly, effective. There were antiacids but no antihistamines.

The whole armamentarium of the physician at that time was very limited. The main thing the doctor wanted to do was to do no harm. If I couldn't do any good, at least I didn't want to do any harm as I judged that some doctors occasionally did.

A doctor who had preceded me in practice in Eclectic had had three or four deaths among women who had delivered babies during the winter of 1932, as I judged because of mismanagement. So I tried very hard to do no harm. I delivered babies without the help of another doctor or a nurse, often in the homes. And not all of these were routine deliveries. I delivered babies with forceps, did versions and extractions, and performed other complicated deliveries. Fortunately the women and most of the babies survived, but it was a horrifying experience to have to do such a raw accouchement.

The people of Eclectic needed a doctor though neither they nor I had any money. They were willing to accept the help of a doctor who was not quite dry behind the ears but was anxious to try to help people. I had many many interesting experiences and learned many things while I lived in Eclectic from the beginning of 1933 until the summer of 1935. I delivered many babies, treated many people with serious illnesses and injuries as well as many with not-so-serious injuries.

For instance, one woman I was called to look after while she was having a baby lived in a one-room house which was across a creek from the nearest road. So I parked my car and walked the footlog across the creek. When I finally arrived at the house, I found a young woman in active labor being "attended" by her mother. The mother had taken a pair of the father-to-be's shoes and placed them under the bed "to control the pain." Hours later, while the young woman continued her labor, her mother-in-law appeared. The mother-in-law, quickly assessing the situation, reached under the bed, picked up the shoes and turned them around 180 degrees and said emphatically, "Some idiot has put these shoes under the bed in the wrong direction! That girl would never have had that baby with the shoes pointed the wrong way!"

Sure enough, the next morning at daylight the baby was born. Then the father caught a chicken on the yard, picked it, fried it, then baked a pan of biscuits in the same frying pan, for it was the only cooking utensil they owned. I shared the meal with the family because during the night rain had swollen the creek, making the footlog impassable until the creek had subsided a bit. Only then was I able to return to my car and drive back to town.

It was also during the worst of the depression (1933) that I was called upon to attend a young woman with acute asthma. Her brother had summoned me and subsequently paid the charges for my visit to his sister, the only time I ever remember a brother paying me for his sister's medical services.

Later that year I delivered a baby (their first) for that same man and his wife in a house so full of holes in the roof that as I sat awaiting the delivery, I could recognize constellations, not individual stars through the roof. After the baby was born, the man rummaged through a trunk and brought out three five-dollar bills to pay me. I would not have taken them had it not been that I owed more people than I didn't owe.

Incidentally, during the re-arming of America, before and during World War II, this man became an earthmover and acquired a fleet of trucks. He was so successful that he later became the outstanding automobile dealer of Montgomery.

I had been in Eclectic maybe ten minutes, having moved down there on a rainy night, when a man came up and asked me if I wasn't the new doctor. I said I was brand new. He said, "Well, I want you to come in here and look at my arm; it's critical."

So he went into what was going to be my office and took off his shirt. Sure enough he had shingles which extended from the middle of his neck down to his finger tips. I was greatly relieved because my very first patient had a diagnosis which I could easily discern. We had no good treatment for shingles (which we still don't have), but the disease was somewhat manageable so I gave thanks unto the Lord silently for those blessings. I told him he had shingles or herpes zoster and prescribed medicine to cover the lesions, another for pain, and a shot of pituitary extract which was thought of in those days as being beneficial for herpes. After I had written down all of these directions, he turned to me and asked, "Doctor, what causes this?" I had to admit that we didn't know what caused herpes. He looked at me in astonishment and asked, "Well, ain't you a doctor?" I admitted that I was but still didn't know what caused herpes. When it was discovered about twenty-five years later that the virus which causes chicken pox causes shingles, I wrote the man a letter telling him I now knew what caused shingles. Incidentally, the next morning the man's wife came to my office and said I had to come right away to see Edison. When I arrived at the old railroad station where they lived, I found Edison broken out with chicken pox. The wife had described him as having "the shingles all over him," so I should have known clinically that the virus causing shingles and that causing chicken pox were closely related, but that didn't occur to me at the time.

One Armistice Day a man came into my office with a cut on the top of his head from being hit in the head with a brick. He was wearing a straw hat, so I very carefully shaved all around the cut, put a sterile glove on my hand, and felt down in the cut to see if there was any piece of straw in the wound. I felt none, so I sewed it up but it didn't heal. I knew there must be some straw in it, so finally I reopened the wound and found a piece of straw as big as a half dollar. If I hadn't searched diligently for it earlier, I wouldn't have felt so badly, but I was embarrassed to realize that I had not been able to feel a piece of straw that large.

Once a man came to me and asked me to go to his house to see his son who had a hurt leg. I found the young man drunk and lying in a typical position with his knee turned in and his foot turned out and his knee partly flexed. He had come from Wewahitchka, Florida, in this condition lying on a mattress in the back of a T-model pickup. His hip had been dislocated for about three days when he arrived in Eclectic. By good luck we were able to replace his hip, and he regained his ability to move about. That fall I was paid three gallons of syrup.

There were many things hard to believe about practicing medicine in a tiny town with no hospital and no x ray machine. The nearest hospital (which was primitive) was fifteen miles away, and Montgomery was thirty miles distant. I had no other doctor whom I could consult because there was jealousy between the two doctors of the town.

Among the other unusual things I experienced in Eclectic was taking out a young man's eye after his eyeball had been ruptured in an accident. I removed the rest of his eyeball and fitted him with a glass eye.

My range of surgery has been from obstetrician and general surgeon to doing mastoidectomies and many tonsilectomies. A surgeon in those days did all kinds of operations.

One of the more pleasant things I ran into in Eclectic was a man named George Shelton. George was a born mechanic who could take an automobile and break it down into its most elementary parts and fix any part of it from the woodwork to the engine or any other part. I delivered a baby for George's wife in December of 1933.

There is a portion of southwest Tallapoosa County which is commonly known as the Corner. It is southwest of Lake Martin and surrounded by Coosa County and the lake; thus it is accessible only by water or through Coosa County via Equality. Many years ago (sometime in the late 1930s) in the Corner, I was treating an old man named Woods for pneumonia with the brand-new sulfonamides. The weather had turned very rainy, and when I got to Equality I found the road impassable. Fortunately, a man who was attending a meeting in progress at the hardshell Baptist Church in Equality had seen me try unsuccessfully to get down the road in my car. He left the church meeting and offered to lend me his horse to ride from Equality to Old Man Woods's house. The man said I would have time to make my call and return while he was in church. Incidentally, Old Man Woods recovered from pneumonia thanks to the sulfonamides, not to my riding the horse. That was the only horse-conveyed trip I made during my practice of medicine.

Another man who lived in Eclectic was a semi-pro veterinarian. He was charged in court with having practiced veterinary medicine without a license and turned loose on probation. He decided to continue his practice, but thereafter if he was called upon to go see a sick animal, he circumvented the law by buying the animal. Then he could legally do anything he wished because the animal was his. This man was Adolphus Moore. One day Adolphus's house caught fire. The telephone operator quickly called around town and reported the fire. People rushed to his house and carried out all the furniture including a hot stove on which his wife was cooking supper. Then they put out the fire with water from his well, and that was the most heroic bit of fire fighting I think I have ever run into.

One of the more unbelievable incidents of my life occurred in Eclectic. If written in fictional form, no one would believe it, but it did happen. One Sunday afternoon I was called to attend a woman who was going to have a baby. I spent the afternoon at the home a couple of miles from town. During the afternoon the woman's brother-in-law walked up noticeably agitated. Two or three days after the baby was born, I checked on her again and she was doing fine. When the baby was about two weeks old, the mother came to my office to give me the baby's name so I could fill out the birth certificate. She confided in me that the baby's name might be in doubt because her husband was not the father of the child. I asked if the father were her husband's brother, and she admitted that he was and thought his name should go on the birth certificate. I explained that in Alabama a woman's husband's name must go on the birth certificate as the father whether he was in fact the father or not. We filled the certificate out that way. After a couple of days, the husband came and paid the bill but said he surely did hate to have to pay it. I asked if he didn't think I had earned my pay by attending his wife during her pregnancy and delivery. He agreed that I had earned my pay, but then he explained, "My wife just hasn't done me right. She was married to another man in Texas, and I bought her a divorce from him. But before she got back to Alabama, she married another man in Texas and then I had to buy a divorce from him. Now she's married me and had the baby, but she's left me and gone to live with Pa."

It was while I lived at Eclectic that I built a sailboat in the back yard by working on it at night. It was a very modest boat only approximately twelve or thirteen feet long of lap strake construction. I carved the mast out of a long piece of lumber and put it all together. You could buy cypress lumber for an unbelievably low price of about $125 for one thousand board feet. Since I needed less than half that amount, sewed the sails myself, and made the gaff, rudder, and seats, the whole thing cost me less than one hundred dollars. Of course, it took a lot of time, but it was a work of love. That was the first sailboat on Lake Martin which in those days was a hog wallow as far as clarity was concerned. There was a great deal of row crop farming around the periphery of the lake, and each time it rained, a lot of soil washed into the lake and muddied it up very badly. In fact, the lake had never cleared up since the dam had been completed several years before. At no time could you see your hand if it was under six inches of water. But I did have a sailboat on Lake Martin in 1933 or 1934.

I also tried my hand at amateur radio for a while in Eclectic. I bought a code machine and a very simple receiver for a total of about $20 and listened to radio with a very elementary single-wire antenna about sixty feet long. And that was my experience with radio in the 1930s.

9

'You Fried the Wrong Egg'

THE LITTLE TOWN OF ECLECTIC WAS FULL OF characters.One of these was "Miss" Annie Williams, a widow who ran the hotel. She was short of statue, about seventy-five years old, and wrinkled like a prune, but had a loud voice with which she did not hesitate to tell anyone how she felt about any subject at any time. Thus her feelings were not carried on her sleeve, but on the air of Eclectic. She took a liking to me and was not only kind in her treatment of me but very helpful in referring patients to me. For instance, through her kindness, I occupied the one room in the hotel with a lavatory. However, there was only cold water available, so I shaved in cold water in the mornings and took my baths across the street in the barber shop.

'Miss' Annie Williams and O. C. Johnson

"Miss Annie" and her brother, O. C. Johnson, lived in the hotel. O. C. was a man of little education but an excellent brain who actually showed signs of having more sense than the President of the United States on occasions. For instance, he would not plow up cotton when farmers didn't have enough shirts to wear or pillows, pillowcases, or sheets. He said he wouldn't plow up cotton when the cotton was needed. Then came the time for the killing of the pigs, a desperate measure in 1933 to bring up the price of pork. But O. C. didn't believe in killing pigs when people on his farm didn't have enough to eat. The authorities gave him a hard time for not obeying these edicts, but he still refused.

Also living in the hotel were Willie Clyde Johnson, the son of O. C., and the mail carrier and his much younger wife. One thing I remember about the mail carrier's wife was that she had ingrown great toenails. So she came to me to have them cut out, a job which I undertook in my office. She had just returned to the hotel when she decided to make a visit to the outhouse. As she walked across the yard, the cow which was in the garden walked over and stepped on her toe which had just been operated on. I think we heard her screaming down at my office.

Some traveling men also came to stay at the hotel on a regular basis. One thing I remember was that we ate quail about three times a week during hunting season because the mail carrier, O. C., and Willie Clyde were all excellent shots.

For amusement we listened to the radio which was downstairs in the parlor where the hot stove was and where people gathered after the evening meal.

After I left Eclectic, Miss Annie came to Alex City to be treated, and I think she died up here in the hospital when she was in her middle eighties. Anybody who said anything unkind about me had spoken unkindly to Miss Annie; she took up for me on all occasions.

The Mayor and the Hardware Store Owner

The mayor had his business only a few houses from the hotel. Although this man was plenty smart and was apparently a good businessman, he could neither read nor write.

Across the street was the town's most famous dope addict, the hardware store owner. He came to his store at about 3:00 a.m. each day, took a big jolt of morphine, and then walked up and down the street singing at the top of his voice. But he had every piece of hardware anyone could imagine, and people came from miles around to buy at this store.

Mr. Hornsby

Diagonally across the street from the hotel was the bank run by Mr. Hornsby, a banker of the old school. By six o'clock every morning, he had swept out the bank and built fires in the fireplaces; then he walked up and down the street looking for people to whom to lend money. He closed the bank promptly at dark every evening.

Dr. Owsley

Dr. Owsley, the doctor who had been shot in Eclectic, qualifies as another of the town's characters. Dr. Owsley had several dope addicts as his patients and would tell the pharmacist to furnish these addicts with dope and not write a prescription for it. Later when he refused to write a prescription, the pharmacist was about to be in real trouble. Thus the pharmacist took out his pistol and shot the doctor five times. However, before the pharmacist came to trial for this deed (good or bad, depending on how you view it), his appendix ruptured and he succumbed to the peritonitis.

Freeman Fincher and Roscoe Wyman

Besides the pharmacist who had shot Dr. Owsley, the other pharmacist in town was Freeman Fincher who had run a drug store in Eclectic for many years. Freeman had a man named Roscoe Wyman working for him, but when Freeman was unable to pay Roscoe, Roscoe finally took over the store and Freeman worked for him until Roscoe owed Freeman so much that he gave the store back to Freeman. They swapped ownership of the drugstore thus several times because neither had money to pay the other.

Big Cat Smith

Another town character was Big Cat Smith, a carpenter who did a good deal of fighting on the weekends. I once sewed up Big Cat's throat from side to side where someone had slit it open.

Wood Fuller

Another unusual character in Eclectic was Wood Fuller. Wood was a cotton buyer and warehouseman. He hung around town from early morning until nearly dark; then he'd look around and say, "Well, it's about dark now. I'm going home and if my supper's not ready I'm going to raise hell, and if it is I'm not going to eat a damn bite." It was also said of him that one morning when his wife had fried his egg, he looked at it in disgust and told her that that was the very time he wanted his egg scrambled. The next morning she served him scrambled egg, but that morning he said he wanted his egg fried. The third morning she fried one egg and scrambled another. He pushed the plate away and commented, "You fried the wrong egg!" That was the kind of reputation he had among the townspeople whether it was deserved or not.

Mr. Thomas

Mr. Thomas also lived in Eclectic. One of his sons was Alexander City's postmaster at one time; another was an astute businessman, but his third son was a ne'er-do-well. This son was a prison guard most of the time and was not the apple of his father's eye. Mr. Thomas, who was diabetic and toothless, spoke of his youngest son this way: "My son Lew-with is the sorriest boy I ever saw that didn't smoke cigarettes."

Dr. Justice

We had an old doctor at Central named Dr. Oscar Justice who was the first doctor in this area to have attended medical school. The other doctors in the area had simply read medicine under some older practitioner and then started practicing. He was quite a character in many ways; he was three times a widower, bought liquor by the ten-gallon keg, and kept a mistress (so the tale was told) when he was seventy-five years old. He took me under his wing for some real education when I moved to Eclectic in 1932. He frequently phoned me to come by his home and go with him to see sick people.

One day we were on our way to see a patient when our car broke down about a mile and a half west of Santuck. While we were standing in the road puzzling over what was the matter with the car, a giant airship came over us. It was either the *Macon* or the *Akron* on its trip across the United States. Dr. Justice looked up at this airship nearly one thousand feet long floating through the sky with eight engines running and said, "What in the world is that?" I told him that I had read that the airship was scheduled to pass over us that day. He looked back down at the car and said, " Well, they ain't no such damn thing as that!" And that was the end of it as far as he was concerned.

After we got the car fixed, he took me to see an old woman of ninety-six years who lived near nearby. When I could find no recognizable syndrome except extreme old age, he asked me what he must put on the death certificate when she died. I replied that senility was the cause, I supposed, since I found nothing else wrong with the woman.

"Oh, no," he replied. "That is not a certifiable cause of death in Alabama."

When I asked what he proposed, he quickly answered, "I'll put down one they'll accept: childbirth!"

Speaking of Dr. Justice, I must tell another unusual thing about him. He didn't believe in paying his bills until the end of the year, and in the first week of the new year he paid up all his bills including those to the power company, the telephone company, the people who supplied him with medicines, and others. If someone came along who demanded that he pay by the month, he promptly told them he was a member of the state senate and he'd see if he couldn't get some better regulations on that type of business in that they were so anxious to collect. He cited that people paid him only in the fall after they had sold their crops, so he thought it was only fair that he pay others after he had been paid. And he did pay all his bills, but he waited as he said according to the Chinese custom of paying only at the first of the year.

10

'She's a Mighty Fine Woman, They Say'

IN JANUARY 1936 GRANNY AND I MOVED TO ALEXANDER City. Using a very modest-sized truck because we didn't have a lot of furniture, we moved into a house in the Lake Hills area owned by Mr. Tom Russell. We paid either fifteen or seventeen dollars a month rent, including electricity and water. It was a modest house with two bedrooms, a living room, dining room, kitchen, and bathroom on its main floor.

Dr. Farrior, my old college friend, had been practicing medicine in Alexander City for several years, but he decided to return to school to specialize and offered me the opportunity to take over his office and his practice. He was my benefactor not only in this way but also in giving me some very good clues to people around town. One man he said was "salt of the earth," that whatever he told me could be relied on to be perfectly honest and honorable. I found him that way too. He told me about other people and some of their peculiarities, and his assessments were exactly correct. Of another man he said, "He's been everywhere, seen everything, and he didn't like it." And that was an exact thumbnail description of the man, who later destroyed himself. The idea of having an established practice was certainly a help. Many of Farrior's patients stuck with me after Farrior left.

Dr. Denney was well-established here, too. He was the company physician for Avondale Mills, and he had quite a practice including lots of surgery. In my early days here, he often used me as his assistant in surgery. I would get about twenty-five dollars as an assistant's fee for major surgery, but that was a payment for a car in those days. So I earned my car payments by assisting in surgery. I had to borrow money to buy a couple of cars because I didn't have enough cash to buy one, but I learned early on that buying on credit was an expensive way to buy an automobile.

About closing time one day, a man came running up to my office very excitedly and told me he wanted me to come to see his pa who was bleeding badly from the nose. I went back in the office and got some nose packing material, a nasal speculum, forceps, flashlight, and a head mirror; then I hurried out past Sanford Bridge to see about "Pa." When I arrived, Pa was sitting on the front porch with a basin in his lap, and his nose was bleeding profusely. He was simply catching the blood to keep from making a mess, but he was getting weaker by the minute. When I looked at his nose, I discovered that the blood wasn't coming from inside his nose but from the nasal labial fold. He had fallen and cut an artery in his face right at the place where the nose joins the face.

All the things I had brought with me way up to Sanford Bridge (approximately twelve miles from Alex City) were materials for stopping a nosebleed from inside the nose, and I was totally unprepared for this situation. There wasn't but one thing I could do: get someone to hold a pack on this bleeding artery until I could prepare some sewing material and sew his face up. But at first I was at a loss for a needle. Finally I found among the "souvenirs" in my bag a curved needle which I had to have for sewing in that particular location; then I didn't have any suture material, so I borrowed some silk from the man's wife and sewed up the man's face without any anesthesia. But I did stop him from bleeding which was a minor triumph as far as I was concerned.

Soon after I moved to Alexander City, I became the doctor for the Tinsley family of Coosa County. There were ten or eleven children in the Tinsley family, but there were no grandchildren though the children were grown and married. Times were hard, and it was difficult to make a living scratching in the hardpan dirt of Coosa County, and the Tinsley's children had decided they didn't need children. But then they decided to increase the population of the earth some, and in one year I delivered either nine or ten babies for various members of this family. One girl had married late in life and had no children; then, with the very last egg she ever matured, she conceived. She realized that this was her very last chance to have a child, so she was very meticulous in her behavior during the pregnancy. She did deliver a baby when she was about forty-eight years old. I think she is the oldest woman I ever delivered a child for, with one possible exception. The child was born in a house in Coosa County in which there was one book, a Sears Roebuck catalog. There was no Bible in the house, but there was the Sears catalog; thus we named the baby "Sears Roebuck."

There are many interesting things that do happen to country doctors. I once had a woman bring her child to me to have her tonsils out. After examining the child, I agreed that the tonsils needed to come out. I did the necessary blood work and urine analysis, and as a last-minute instruction, the mother said to me, "Be sure and cut out that thing that hangs down the middle of her throat."

I looked at her and asked, "Do you mean the uvula, the little trigger device that hangs down the back of the throat?"

"Yes," she answered. "Dr. ____ removed mine."

Now the uvula separates things which go to the esophagus from those which go into the trachea, so in spite of her instructions, I was careful not to remove the uvula when I did the tonsillectomy on the child.

Soon after I came to Alex City, Dr. J. A. M. Nolen came to me and said there was a child up above Hackneyville who needed attention. He had seen the child and believed she had appendicitis and needed to be operated on. He asked me if I would perform the surgery. In a moment of weakness, I agreed to operate if I thought the child needed surgery. I went to see the child, whose name was Mae West, of all things. The child did have acute appendicitis, the family had no money, and the situation was very bad all around. Dr. Nolen agreed to put the child to sleep, if I'd take out her appendix. So we came back to town and got some instruments and a sterilized linen pack, and went back to the house. Out in the yard, under the shade of an oak tree, in daylight, I took out the child's appendix while Dr. Nolen gave the anesthetic and shooed the flies away.

Even more unbelievable, right here in Alex City a local dry cleaning man had two daughters who were registered nurses. They were good nurses, but they didn't trust what went on at the hospital at the time. So when their father had a bilateral inguinal hernia, they wanted to have it repaired for him at home. They prepared things at their home on Lafayette Street, and with the patient under general anesthesia, while Dr. Walls repaired one hernia, I repaired the other.

One reason people didn't trust their loved ones to the hospital unless they absolutely had to was that in 1941 there was only one woman, a Mrs. Betts, on duty at night in Russell Hospital. Mrs. Betts had studied nursing by correspondence. Not only was she the nurse, but she answered the telephone and fired the boiler on cold nights. She was a woman for all seasons!

I also helped Dr. Street remove a Mr. Dark's appendix at his home near Kellyton because again the family didn't trust the hospital.

I once nailed a man's hip in my office. This occurred in about 1949. This black man who lived near Cottage Grove had sustained a fall. His family had taken Venetian blind tape about two inches wide and made a spica (a homemade cast of overlapping spiral bandage to immobilize a limb) of it in which they wrapped the man's leg from his pelvis to his heel. Then they had brought him in the bed of a truck to my office. He told me that he would either have to lie in that spica and hope to get well, or I could do something for him in my office. But he didn't have money to go to a hospital, and he refused to take charity. I took the man into my office, and using spinal anesthesia, Mrs. Pickens (my nurse at the time) and I proceeded to nail up his hip under the guidance of occasional x-ray pictures. (I had had some training at Harvard in advanced orthopedics.) The man walked again and walked for many years, thanks largely to his fortitude in withstanding such treatment.

Once I was doing rectal surgery on a woman in my office, and under the influence of medication for pain and anxiety, the patient was hallucinating. Now Miss Bessie Hawkins ran a beauty parlor across the hall. Miss Bessie was a talker, and at this particular time, she was walking up and down the hall talking incessantly. The patient who was hallucinating called out, "Somebody cut off that talking machine out there! I can't stand to hear that thing talk any more!"

Speaking of things which were done in the office, there were many years when Drs. Street, Walls, Denney, and I removed people's tonsils in our offices. We were pretty well equipped for such things. I took out Sandy Petrey's tonsils and my oldest daughter Chick's tonsils the same day in my office, kept them there all day, and then took them home that night. Occasionally, when we had complications, we would stay with the patient in the office overnight, but we were equipped for that too with two or three beds. But ordinarily we let them go home about sundown.

Among other almost unbelievable things which happened to me, one day as I was walking out of the hospital, a sawyer walked up to me holding his belly and said, “It’s done et through.” When I asked what he meant, he said that he had an ulcer in his stomach and that it had eaten through. Sure enough when I took him inside and examined him, I found that he had a perforated peptic ulcer. He recovered and is still living today as far as I know. That was unusual in that the man made his own diagnosis.

There was a registered nurse in town who had married late in life and was pregnant with her only child. One night about two o’clock, as I was treating another patient at the hospital, she came in and told me something terrible had happened to her. An examination showed that she was the victim of uterine apoplexy, abruptio placenta. That is the placenta had separated from the womb, bleeding was taking place within the womb, and she was about to die. But she was smart enough and well-educated enough in medicine to know that something was horribly wrong. And she had come to seek help without waiting for a doctor to come to her first. The upshot was that she had to have blood transfusions and a hysterectomy in addition to a Caesarean section. She is still alive and was made Woman of the Year here in Alexander City a few years ago.

After the law was enacted about 1938 requiring premarital examination of the groom to certify that the man was free of venereal disease, a man about seventy-five years old came to my office requesting such clearance. When I asked him where he lived, he replied that he lived in the county home near Jackson’s Gap. The “county home” was a euphemism for almshouse. Out of curiosity I asked him who was the prospective bride? He said, “She’s a lady living in the home with me. And they say she’s a mighty fine woman.”

Twelve miles from Eclectic is Equality. One morning I was called to Equality to tend a childbirth and was told to hurry. When I arrived, I met for the first time a Mr. and Mrs. Parker and their daughter who was about to deliver her second baby. The daughter’s husband had been afflicted with a malignancy while she was carrying this baby and had died from a sarcoma of some sort. She had planned to go to Montgomery for the baby's delivery and had been there for prenatal care, but she had awakened in the middle of the night in labor and unable to travel to Montgomery. So they had called me. I delivered the baby and thus met the Parkers and their daughter who were wonderful people and later became our close friends. The daughter later married a man with whom I had grown up in Birmingham. During the war he had been a prisoner of war in the Philippines; after the war he had returned to Alabama and married his now-widowed childhood sweetheart. They live down in Jacksonville, Florida, and have two grown children of their own. We occasionally still hear from them. Mrs. Parker lived into her nineties and was always a most pleasant woman. It was a pleasure to have been called in such an emergency and meet such nice people under such harrowing circumstances.

Everything was not so pleasant nor funny in medicine. In the early 1920s,'30s, and '40s, there were company doctors for both Russell and Avondale Mills in Alexander City. Dr. Denney was the company doctor for Avondale, and Dr. Chapman was the Russell Company doctor. These doctors were salaried, and they were treated with little respect by many of their clientele. The fact that the workers were paying a pittance each month for a doctor made the people most inconsiderate of the doctor in many cases. When Dr. Chapman or Dr. Denney went on a vacation, I would fill in for them. I remember being called to a house about seven o'clock one morning and being told that it was an emergency. When I arrived, I found that the emergency was that the people had to be at work by eight o'clock, so they had decided to get the doctoring done before work. Another time I went to see a sick child only to have the mother go out on the back porch and call in a loud voice, "Johnny, come home from that ball game. The doctor is here to see you." Incidents such as these were the result of the people being required by their employer to pay for medical services. They felt that they were paying for medical care, and they were determined to get it. Yet while these incidents were inconsiderate of the doctor, still other incidents which occurred in one of the mill villages were enough to bring tears to my eyes. Once I went into the family bathroom to wash my hands only to find coal stored in the bathtub for the winter; certainly no one was going to use the tub before warm weather. Another time I treated a child with pneumonia whose long underwear had to be cut off because he had been "sewed in for the winter."

Certainly every doctor gains some medical knowledge outside of medical schools. For instance, I learned that postpartal hemorrhage can often be stopped by putting the baby to the mother's breast! This was taught me by a midwife in the backwoods where no oxytocic drug was available. A midwife also taught me that ice-cold water given a woman with uterine inertia will speed up the second stage of labor in a dramatic fashion. From a farmer I learned that soot from the fireplace will help stop bleeding as well as oxycel or some more esoteric products.

He is now a college professor, but then he was only a ten-year-old boy with tonsils which had given him a lot of trouble. It was decided that his tonsils should be removed. Well, his father and mother decided that he should also have another operation at the same time, an operation which is usually done on a male infant, traditionally about the eighth or tenth day of life and today sometimes performed before the baby leaves the hospital after his birth. Dr. Denney did one operation, and I did the other. The little boy recovered, and when he had regained his voice, he told his baby sister, "Your tonsils ain't where you think they are."

Many years ago, I went back to Birmingham to learn more about infant feeding from my good friend Dr. Wallace Clyde. While there, I stayed with Pop Menefee whose wife was on a trip to Europe.

One morning the phone rang with a request for Pop to stop by the home of Melissa, the Menefees' cook, who had been out sick for several weeks. When we stopped at Melissa's, we found her lying in bed but furious. She reached under her pillow, brought out a Birmingham newspaper, and showed Pop an article saying that Felix (her husband) had married.

She said, "I just want you to look here and see what Felix done while I was sick in the hospital. He has done got hisself couthouse married to that sorry Donie! I knowed he'd been in bed with her for two years, but now while I was sick in the bed, he done got hisself couthouse married to her!"

Pop said, "Well, I'm sorry, Melissa, but what is it you want me to do?"

She said she wanted him to send the sheriff to her house so she could swear out a warrant against Felix for bigamy. She said, " I want him put under the jail and kept there." Then she added, "I ought to take out my double-bladed axe and cut his head off. Here he's been snoring in my face and eating my cornbread; then when I get sick, he goes off and marries that sorry Donie!"

Pop agreed to send the sheriff but warned her he was not going to get Felix out of jail when he was arrested.

Melissa assured Pop she wanted Felix never to get out but to stay in jail for the rest of his life.

The upshot of the incident was that the sheriff did arrest Felix for bigamy. When his trial came up, Mrs. Menefee and a couple of her friends went to the courthouse to listen to the proceedings and offer moral support to Melissa. Just before the appointed hour, Melissa came up and informed Mrs. Menefee that there wasn't going to be a trial because they had settled out of court.

Melissa explained, "Felix agreed to pay my doctor bill and my hospital bill and we's done settled out o' cout." She looked around surreptitiously and added, "And, besides, I just happened to remember, I got two other livin' husbands."

11

No Car to Go to a Funeral

WHILE ECLECTIC HAD ITS SHARE, OR PERHAPS A few more than its share of eccentric characters, there were some in Alex City who are worthy of mention. Some were very serious, some comical, and some hilariously funny.

John Orphan

One of the serious ones was a restaurateur, John Orphan who ran the Climax Cafe on Main Street. He ran an excellent cafe. He had a few eccentricities, but not many. John was born on the island of Corfu, came to America as a small boy, and was in San Francisco during the 1906 earthquake and fire. So he had been an American before I was (I was not born until 1907). John often told me that I was an interloper, and this was his country; we often joked and had fun about that.

John was a good citizen who took part in any charitable or social event when he was called upon. He ran a good cafe in which you could get a nice t-bone steak for seventy-five cents or a vegetable lunch for thirty-five cents and a lunch with meat for forty-five cents. Before I was married, John would sometimes ask me to come have supper with him. He would always have some special dish which he may have cooked himself or might have had his excellent cook, Murphy, prepare. We would often share squid or fresh shrimp, and I greatly appreciated his kindness.

Dwight Craig

There was another town character named Dwight Craig, who had suffered a very serious and most peculiar illness. He had an abcess around one kidney which ate through his diaphragm, causing him to have an inflamation of his pleura on that side. The abcess of the pleura broke into a bronchus, and the fellow spat up urine for several weeks. He's the only patient I ever saw who spat up urine. Furthermore, I have talked to several urologists, none of whom had ever had a patient with these symptoms.

But when we opened up his side, drained the pus, and formed another way for it to get out of his body, he stopped coughing on the operating table and had an almost miraculous recovery. This illness, however, did partially affect his mind. He would stand on the street corner and as people passed, he would call their names and make some poignant comment about them such as where they were from, when they came to Alex City, or what they did for a living. For instance, one man he talked about was the police chief about whom he made very unkind comments; he was also unkind in his comments about Cal Alison. Cal was a fine young man from Selma who had come to Alex City and married Mr. Ben Russell's daughter.

Though Cal was a very nice young man, Dwight always dwelled on the fact that he was a school teacher who had married a rich man's daughter and now was a big shot. Cal never considered himself a big shot that I know of, but Dwight had him pegged that way. Dwight spoke of another man by saying he was a son of so-and-so, born and raised in Alexander City, a big shot, and had a weak mind. He made some most unkind comments about others too. Well, I didn't want him telling folks the bare truth about me, so occasionally I would go in John Orphan's cafe and give him a dollar to buy Dwight a good meal when he would come in. Both men appreciated this, and Dwight never said bad things about me which he easily could have. Thus Dwight Craig was my friend all the time.

Sanford Mullins

Another character who was well-known over the state was Sanford Mullins. He was a lawyer and politician who had served in the legislature.

But Sanford was primarily a raconteur; he could tell stories better than anyone else I ever ran into. He had been at one time the private secretary to Senator Tom Heflin from whom he had supposedly learned the art of tale-telling. Stories which were hilarious when he told them were not nearly so funny when I recounted them.

Methodists

After Edith and I had been married for a few years and lived on Greene Street, we had a preacher at the First Methodist Church who preached in such a loud voice that I could sit on our front porch about 175 yards away and hear him. I guess he thought the Lord was deaf.

Speaking of churches, once a year at the Methodist Church was layman's Sunday and one of the laymen of the church delivered the message. One such layman, though he was an outstanding citizen with lots of ability and a good heart, had not had much schooling. He thought we didn't fully appreciate the wonderful voice of Mrs. Catherine Thomas, the lead soprano in the choir of that time. In fact, he said, "Mrs. Catherine has a better voice than any of those Eyetalian or Oriental opera singers."

On another occasion, the same man as part of his sermon was telling about a book he had read by a man named Melville. (I'm sure he hadn't read a library full of books in his whole life.) In this book, said the storyteller, a sailor from New England went whaling in the South Seas. While whaling, he had an accident in which he lost a leg and blamed it all on a white whale. After he recovered, he returned to the South Seas and was out to get revenge on the whale. Finally spotting the whale, he called out the long boats; his men rowed hard, and as they approached the whale, Captain Ahab stood up in the front of the boat and "threw the poontang in him."

Mr. Ben

It was my good fortune to have Mr. Ben Russell as a patient. I can't tell much about his private medical history, but I can tell some things about the man in general. He was more or less a fanatic about germs and infection and opened doors with his hand in his coat pocket instead of putting it directly on the door knob. He drank prune juice, celery juice, and raisin juice for health foods long before they became a fad. He also frequented doctors around the country including a doctor in Philadelphia, one in Grand Rapids, Michigan, one in New Orleans, and one in Gadsden, Alabama. Not surprisingly, he was very smart in his choice of doctors and picked out some outstanding ones. He didn't feel that he was going to live a long time, and it was easy to see why. He had aged very quickly and was known as "Old Man Ben" when he was only about forty-five. He lived to be only sixty-four; longevity just wasn't for him. He had rowing machines in his house and was a health fanatic, but he never had very good health.

Mr. Ben was very smart. He was well-educated in several ways and was a very hard worker. He carried every ad and piece of mail which came to him home at night and studied and planned until about midnight every night. He was also dedicated to his business, his church, his fraternity, the universities he had attended, and to educational institutions all over. He was on the boards of directors of the University of Alabama, Howard College, Tuskegee Institute, and the University of Virginia. His abilities were well recognized by a great many people. There are people who deprecate his efforts and remember only the unkind things which must happen to any great man, but as far as I am concerned, he was a really great man.

Mr. Ben died two weeks after Pearl Harbor, but in the year before Pearl Harbor, as America was arming, automobile production stopped with only a very little warning. I had an automobile that had been run only a few thousand miles, but when the handwriting was on the wall that car production was about to stop, I phoned Mr. Ben one morning and asked him what he thought I should do about getting me a new car even though my present one had only three thousand miles. He agreed that the manufacturers were going to stop making cars and that cars would not be available for a good many years. He said, "I can't tell you what you ought to do, but I will tell you that I bought several trucks this morning and had them put in the warehouse."

One other note which may seem completely incongruous to the present generation: Mr. Ben was not only president of the First National Bank, he also had a printing business, a bakery, a dairy, an enormous farm, the Russell Mills, a hotel in North Carolina and one or two in Florida, and a few other business interests around the world. But he picked up the phone himself when you called Number 1 on the Alex City telephone system and said, "Ahem, Ben Russell speaking." He didn't have a secretary to answer the phone for him, but after Mr. Ben had answered, Sam Bradshaw would pick up on an extension and write down the entire conversation for the record. Mr. Ben didn't have a dictation machine, but he had Sam which was exactly the same thing. Thus when Mr. Ben died, Sam knew more about his business than did any of his three sons: Tom, Bennie, or Robert.

R. C. Ray

Another character of the town who died only a few years ago was R. C. Ray. He was a barber with a loud voice in which he often expressed his opinions. R. C. would invite Sanford Mullins and me to his home about once a year to eat collards, backbone, and apple pie. Sanford and I both looked forward to that day.

Dr. Harlan

There have been many doctors in this area who were real characters. One was Dr. Harlan. Known for his short temper, he was also known to have threatened to cut his horse's throat because his horse wouldn't stand still to be saddled. Dr. Harlan did shoot his Hupmobile when it wouldn't start one day!

Mrs. Harlan, as head of the local chapter of the U.D.C, collected money from all sources to afford our town a statue of the Confederate soldier, the statue which for years stood in the public square on Broad Street and which now stands in the city Sportsplex. Her efforts extended to the black community, and when the statue was placed on the public square, many of the solicited blacks thought it was a statue of Dr. Harlan who had coincidentally died only a few months before.

Dr. Foshee

Another character who lived near, though not in Alex City, was Dr. Reuben Foshee who lived at Newsite. Dr. Foshee looked just like Will Rogers, the famous wit, and because of this resemblance attempted to emulate him. He was a country practitioner who made no bones about having started his practice in 1907 riding a Texas pony with saddlebags on each side and a derby hat on his head.

He told about riding through the country and one day coming

upon a place where several people were sitting around outside a house with a dogtrot in the middle and a room on each side. On a cot lay a man who was vomiting into a large tub with newspapers around it. His belly was distended, his face was drawn, and he was feverish. Dr. Foshee, without even removing his hat, looked at the man and said, "Well, it's obvious what the diagnosis is: the man's bowels are locked."

One man sitting by the bedside spoke up, "I ain't no doctor, but his bowels have been moving every twenty minutes."

"Well," Dr. Foshee said, "that's the trouble. They are locked wide open, and that's the worst kind."

Another tale that Dr. Foshee used to tell was about the first January after he had finished school. On a bitterly cold night, he had just gotten in bed when he heard a horse come down the frozen road and pull up under his window.

The rider called out, "Oh, Doc."

"Yes," he said.

The man said, "Pa wants you to come down to the house to see the baby. It's sick and they don't know what to do with it."

Dr. Foshee climbed out of bed, dressed, saddled his horse, and rode down to Germany's Ferry to see the sick baby. He saw the baby but had no idea what was the matter with it. He made out some powders and told the family to give one to the baby every four hours, and with the help of the Lord and the medicine he expected the child to recover. He got back on his horse and rode back home thinking what a wonderful service he had performed for humanity.

He had just gotten back in bed and gotten warm when he heard the same horse coming down the frozen road again. The rider pulled up under his window again and called out, "Oh, Doc!" Dr. Foshee asked what was wrong now. The man replied, "Pa wants you back at the house. Them are twin babies, and they showed you the wrong one."

Dr. Banks lived at Dadeville at the same time Dr. Foshee lived at Newsite; they frequently consulted each other and shared much of the same rural territory. Once when Dr. Foshee went to attend a labor case down near Horseshoe Bend, the woman developed acute eclampsia. Dr. Foshee was horrified and sent the woman's husband, in Dr. Foshee's car, to get Dr. Banks. In a couple of hours, the husband returned without Dr. Banks but with the message that Dr. Banks told him he had been up all night and had to get some sleep. He had sent word to Dr. Foshee to "just control them spells till I get there!"

Once another local doctor handed a man a prescription, and not only did the man not pay the doctor but asked the doctor to loan him the money with which to buy the medicine. The doctor said, "Hand me back that prescription; I put something in it for your nerves, but you don't need anything for your nerves!"

Dr. Chapman's Driver, Simme

When Dr. Chapman was on vacation, his driver, a black man named Simme, drove for me when I made calls in Dr. Chapman's stead. Simme was a great help because he knew where everyone lived, what was wrong with the patients, and how Dr. Chapman was treating them. One day Simme and I drove out to see a Mr. P___ who baffled me with his many complaints. He had Munchausen's syndrome; he was obsessed with fooling doctors. His mantelpiece was filled with medicines he had been prescribed by different doctors. I didn't recognize what was wrong with him, so on the way back to town I asked Simme what Dr. Chapman had been treating Mr. P___ for. He quickly replied, "Oh, that man can take a doctor anytime."

Mack Lauderdale

In thinking of characters in Alexander City, one who stands out is my black friend, Mack Lauderdale, otherwise known as "String," a contraction of "Stringbean." Mack Lauderdale worked for us for many years as kind of a major-domo. He said he raised Jimmy. He was the driver on several occasions and general factotum. He helped me lay brick when we first built our house. I wanted to have some part of that house which I had helped with physically, so with Mack's help I laid the brick sidewalk which runs from the driveway to the front steps. Mack was a man of very limited schooling, but with a very odd vocabulary. He would say that things were "sufficious" or that they would "suit your royal dignity."

Once I wanted to put a self-bailing device into the cabin cruiser which I had built because it always leaked a little bit. So I had the boat up on a trailer cutting a hole in the bottom. Mack came along and saw what I was doing. He asked, "Doctor, what you doin' drilling a hole in the

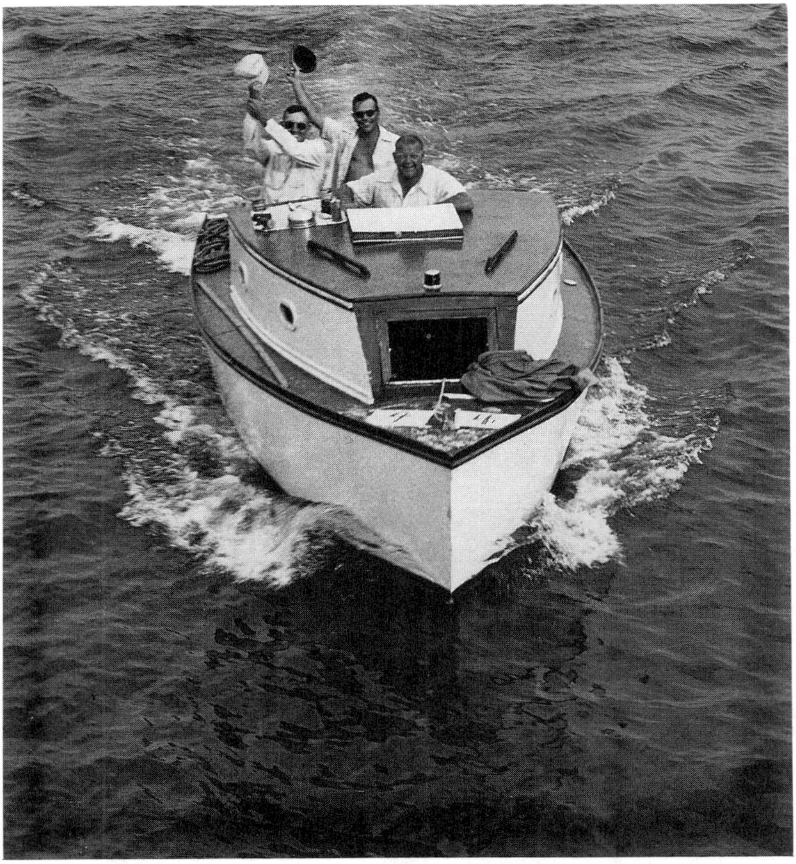

Jim Cameron, Frank Penton, and Hamp Lyon on the cabin cruiser that Jim built, Fourth of July boat race on Lake Martin—1953.

bottom of the boat?"

I said, "Mack, I'm doing that to let the water out."

Obviously disbelieving, he replied, "Yessah, you're gonna make a hole in the bottom of the boat to let the water out."

Well, when I finished the work, I had Mack put on a life preserver and get into the boat with me. I turned off the self-bailer, we launched the boat, started up the engine, and got moving pretty well. Then I opened up the self-bailer, and sure enough, water poured into the bottom of the boat.

Mack looked at the water pouring in and commented, "Yessah, you'se gonna let the water outta the boat."

Then we gained a little more speed, and the self-bailer was activated. The water receded and dried out the bottom of the boat. Mack looked at this bug-eyed, and commented, "We needs one of them on the other side."

My friend Dr. Denney had a pond a little north of Alex City in which he had many fish. He also had a rowboat which leaked pretty badly, so I decided the thing to do was to repair his rowboat. Thus I took Mack to the pond with me one day, and we took the rowboat out of the water and patched it.

While we were up there, I decided to do a little fly fishing. I asked Mack to paddle the boat for me, and he volunteered to go dig some

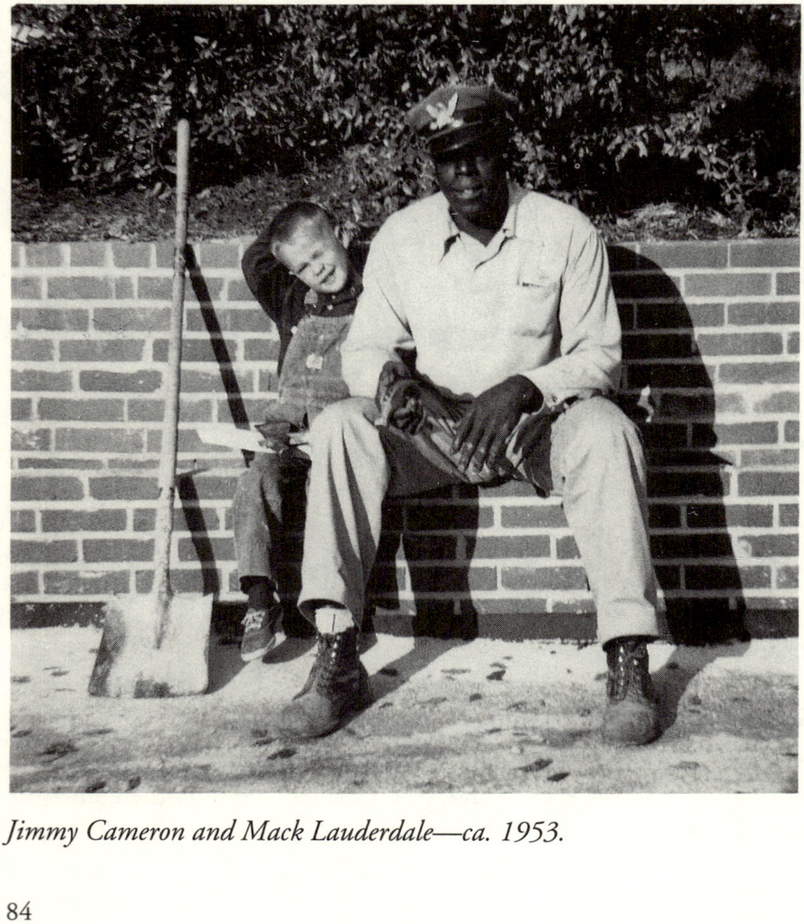

Jimmy Cameron and Mack Lauderdale—ca. 1953.

"baits" for me. I told him I didn't need any bait because I was going to use a fly. While I was rigging up my line, Mack was shaking his head in disbelief and muttering, "You goin' fishing and you ain't goin' take no baits."

Well, it so happened that I had a very lucky streak, and as we went around the lake, I boated several fish.

Mack nearly had a fit every time I would catch one. He kept repeating, "You catchin' fish and ain't using no baits attall. I don't know why other folks ain't caught on yet. They been diggin' them baits all the time."

Yet that wasn't quite as funny as Mack's comments about our cars in 1957. In that year we bought a Volkswagen and and a Corvette, and we still had the station wagon we had bought in 1954 or 1955. Mack said, "You got three automobiles, but you ain't nothing to go to a funeral in!"

Mack built Jimmy a tree house in a big oak tree behind our house on Ridgeway Drive. Mack would get up in the tree house with Jimmy, and they had great times there.

After Jimmy died, Mack was still living and kept dogging me for a picture of Jimmy. But I don't believe I ever gave him that picture because I'd just forget it. Now Mack too has passed on to his reward.

Mr. Proctor

Thinking of Mack Lauderdale reminds me of another handyman who lived far from Alex City.

Mr. Proctor was a man of many talents who was a neighbor of my brother-in-law, Todd Craig, in Falls Church, Virginia. Now Todd was an engineer trained at Rutgers University. One time he wanted to modify his house by installing a fireplace around which heat would circulate. He wanted the cold air to go in at the sides and come out at the top (as many are made to do today).

Mr. Proctor didn't understand this project, and thus he refused to build it the way Todd told him to. He told Todd, "The way you've got this thing designed, it won't work. Air rises."

Todd agreed, "Yes, of course, air rises. Hot air rises and cold air falls. Remember how you can feel the cold air on your feet if you open the refrigerator."

Mr. Proctor insisted, "No, Mr. Craig, air rises."

Finally, in exasperation, Todd told him, "Mr. Proctor, I spent four years in college studying engineering, and I tell you hot air rises, and cold air falls!"

Mr. Proctor's self-satisfied reply was, "Mr. Craig, lotta folks spend four years in college and don't learn anything."

Judge Jack Coley

Before he was Judge Coley, he was just plain Jack Coley and worked at the First National Bank. When we married, I took Edith into the bank and introduced her to Jack. I told him she was my better half, and anything I had in my checking account was hers up to and including four dollars.

Jack's sister Rebecca Heard worked for me for a few years. She was a fairly young widow then, and though she had no secretarial training, she was very faithful about coming to work and was friendly and nice to the people who came into my office which meant a lot. Then she met Mr. Gilbert who had come here to inspect the products made in the local foundry for the City of New York. They married and had a daughter Nanette.

Jack was at the University when I started there. He was an outstanding student there, and after his graduation returned to Alexander City to work in the bank. Then he ran for the office of Probate Judge and was elected after an old politician from Dadeville had held the office for many years. He is a very progressive person. During Jack's term of office, the old court house was replaced by a new one, and he was also very instrumental in having Horseshoe Bend made into a national park. His talents did not go unrecognized when he retired from politics, and he was made president of the Alexander City Bank. In fact, he has just recently retired as the chairman of the board of that bank though he is ninety-four. He is still very active and quick-witted.

Raydeen McKinney

Raydeen worked in the surgery suite of Russell Hospital. But she also sang in a quartet, and she loved to tell about the quartet (there were six of them in the "quartet": five men and Raydeen). According to Raydeen, they could "saing real good." One time the quartet went to

Atlanta to cut a record. For this venture, they were gone from Friday afternoon till Tuesday afternoon. When Raydeen returned to work, I asked her, "Raydeen, your husband went with you to Atlanta, didn't he?"

"Oh, no, sir," she replied, "he can't saing."

Now Raydeen's regular preacher was out of town one time, and so they hired a fill-in preacher. The regular preacher was quite tall, but the substitute was very short. While the substitute was in town, he preached a revival, and after he had preached against gambling, whiskey drinking, card playing, and adultery, he was about out of topics on which to preach. So at the next service, he preached against wearing low-cut dresses.

After the sermon, one of the sisters went to him and said, "You is so different from our regular preacher. He real tall, and you real short. He real black, but you high yellow. But what I really can't understand is why you don't like us wearing these low-cut dresses. Our regular preacher like that. In fact, he sometime put his head on my bosom and say he can hear the angels singin'."

The little short preacher said, "I believe I'll try that. " So he put his head down and listened a minute. Then he said, "I don't hear no angels singing."

The sister responded, "No wonder, you ain't plugged in yet!"

Now when I see Raydeen in the grocery store, I ask, "Raydeen, how are those little, short preachers getting along?"

She still remembers the story too because she says, "They ain't doin' no better."

12

Medical Rewards and Liabilities

FROM THE TIME THAT I BECAME A DOCTOR UNTIL the present time, the world has changed a great deal in the rewards that a doctor gets for practicing medicine. There was a time in the early years of my life when the reward of medicine was accomplishment. Now the reward is money, something entirely different. I'm sure that some of the doctors I knew hardly made a living, but they took great pride in their accomplishments, as much as someone today would take in how much money he or she made.

There was a time when almost no patient had any insurance. There was no such thing as medical or surgical insurance. There were a few institutions which had medical plans which were the equivalent of medical insurance. Employees of companies such as United States Steel in Birmingham and Russell Corporation in Alexander City paid a pittance per week into a medical fund, and for that they could get a doctor to come to their house or could go to the doctor's office to see him. They paid only a very little bit, but they got a very little bit in return.

The change to insurance or the government paying one's medical bill has come about during my lifetime. Within my lifetime too has come a change from a few ineffective drugs that were about as effective as burning feathers or dancing around the bed to the antibiotics, antihistaminics, immunosuppressive drugs, and many advanced types of medication which were undreamed of in 1930 when I first started practicing medicine.

Gone are the days when a blood transfusion was a major process requiring a couple of surgeons (and I did help transfuse blood into an ex-governor of Alabama in 1930 or 1931 along with two of the outstanding surgeons of Birmingham). Now a nurse's assistant can give a transfusion. We also now have heart and lung transplants in which the immunosuppressive drugs are so vital, but we still don't have a cure for the common cold, nor has anybody ever cured a case of rabies. Thus we have a way to go, even at this time.

In the Medical Association of Alabama, of which I was an active member for all of my medical life, we had a dictum that no monetary consideration should ever be discussed in a medical association meeting. That was a written law of the organization. Now most of the medical association business is devoted to dollars and cents, so that has been a complete turnaround. We also had a complete divorcement of politics from medicine for many years. Nobody at the state Medical Association would say we should advocate Joe Jones for governor because he was in favor of such and such acts for medicine. Now we have "political action committees." These political action committees of the state of Alabama, much to my disgust, will appropriate and spend many thousands of dollars to the advancement of two candidates for the same political office.

In my early days of practice in Eclectic, I inherited two elderly patients whom I dearly loved, two doctor patients. They were Dr. Hunter at Equality and Dr. Justice at Central. I had no idea that I shouldn't do everything in the world which I could for these two old men living alone in isolated communities. Central was five miles from Eclectic, and Equality was twelve miles away. Many times I got up at night to go see one or the other of these men, and I thought nothing of it.

I also had the pleasure of treating several other doctors during my years of practice: Dr. Foshee, Dr. Chapman, Dr. Street, Dr. Askin, Dr. Denney, Dr. J. A. M. Nolen, and Dr. I. D. Nolen (at Newsite). In treating these fellow physicians, I never dreamed of charging them a dime for my services. I remember distinctly operating on one doctor's wife and being very happy that she recovered from a very serious surgical emergency. After I finished working on her, I learned that she had some insurance which would pay the doctor some, but I insisted that her husband keep the money. Incidentally, I also had occasion to use doctors myself and for my wife and children to use them. I operated on the children of other doctors, and they operated on mine. I do remember giving one doctor a case of whiskey as a gratuity or gift of love, but as far as paying other doctors money, that simply wasn't done by mutual agreement. It is entirely different now; doctors expect to be paid for what they do. Maybe that is correct, but maybe the other way was better.

Company doctors were much in vogue during the twenties and thirties. People were desperate for money, and through their companies they had a way of paying the doctor by the week. A dollar or dollar and a half per week would cover the cost of medical care for a family. That was everything: delivery of a baby, treatment of a broken leg, pneumonia, or whatever. The workers paid the corporation, and the corporation paid the doctor for his services. Hospital bills were also paid from this fund; however, hospital bills didn't amount to much then. About two dollars per day was the average cost of a bed in a ward, maybe only one dollar for black people. A private room cost perhaps five dollars per day. Dr. Denney worked on the people in Alexander City who worked for Avondale while Dr. Chapman was the Russell company doctor. When either was out of town, I would pinch hit for him and sometimes make as many as twenty or twenty-five house calls in twenty-four hours earning about a dollar and a half per call. At that rate I thought I was doing marvelously well.

Back in 1933 we charged fifteen dollars for delivery of a baby including prenatal and postnatal care until the baby was six weeks old which often entailed going to the home to see about the baby several times. Of course, if the baby had to be circumcised, that was also included. The idea of giving free prenatal care was to encourage women to come to the office for such care; otherwise, many would not come but would skip prenatal care altogether.

Not everything was bad about the situation at all. For instance, the doctor's wife on whom I did emergency surgery was operated on and given a blood transfusion within one hour of the time we first saw her.

At other times, care was not what it should have been. I remember one Saturday afternoon when I had a patient brought into the hospital with placenta previa. She needed an immediate Caesarean section which I did with the aid of only one nurse who had not finished training but who was the only help available at the time. We had to give the woman a spinal anesthetic in spite of her blood loss, but we did manage to save her though the baby had died. However, we felt that saving the mother was something of a therapeutic triumph.

Just last week a man died here in Alexander City at the age of seventy-odd. Many years ago, Dr. Denney and I operated on this man for a ruptured stomach. He had been playing basketball when one of his opponents accidentally (or on purpose) stuck a knee into the area between his ribs and his navel and ruptured his stomach. He must have had a large gas bubble in his stomach to have brought about such a catastrophe. We sewed up this man's stomach, and he lived until just a short time ago. When the man's wife later went to work in the operating room, she realized what a miracle it was that her husband had not died of his injury.

13

Two Worn-Out Automobiles and a House Full of Children

ONE OF THE NICEST THINGS WHICH HAPPENED to me at Eclectic was that I met my future wife. Edith Ellison came to Eclectic to teach school after having finished Huntingdon College in the spring of 1935. I had already started coming to Alex City to practice medicine in the mornings and would practice in Eclectic in the afternoons. Then in January of 1936, I moved to Alexander City but traveled back to Eclectic to see Edith. After that year Edith went to Roanoke to teach for two years, so I traveled to Roanoke to see her. Then she decided not to teach one year, so I had to go to Hurtsboro, her hometown, to date her. Our courtship lasted from 1935 to 1939 before I felt I could afford to marry and persuaded her to marry me. In the meantime, I wore out two automobiles courting her. Until we married on August 1, 1939, we never lived in the same town except for those few months in Eclectic. Strangely enough for present times, we are still living together.

Our wedding took place at her mother's home in Hurtsboro. Her mother put on a beautiful wedding for us with all the trimmings, and a few of our friends from Alexander City came down there to the wedding ceremony and reception.

Our wedding trip was to Biloxi, Mississippi, and on to San Antonio and Austin, Texas. When we returned home, I took my bride over the

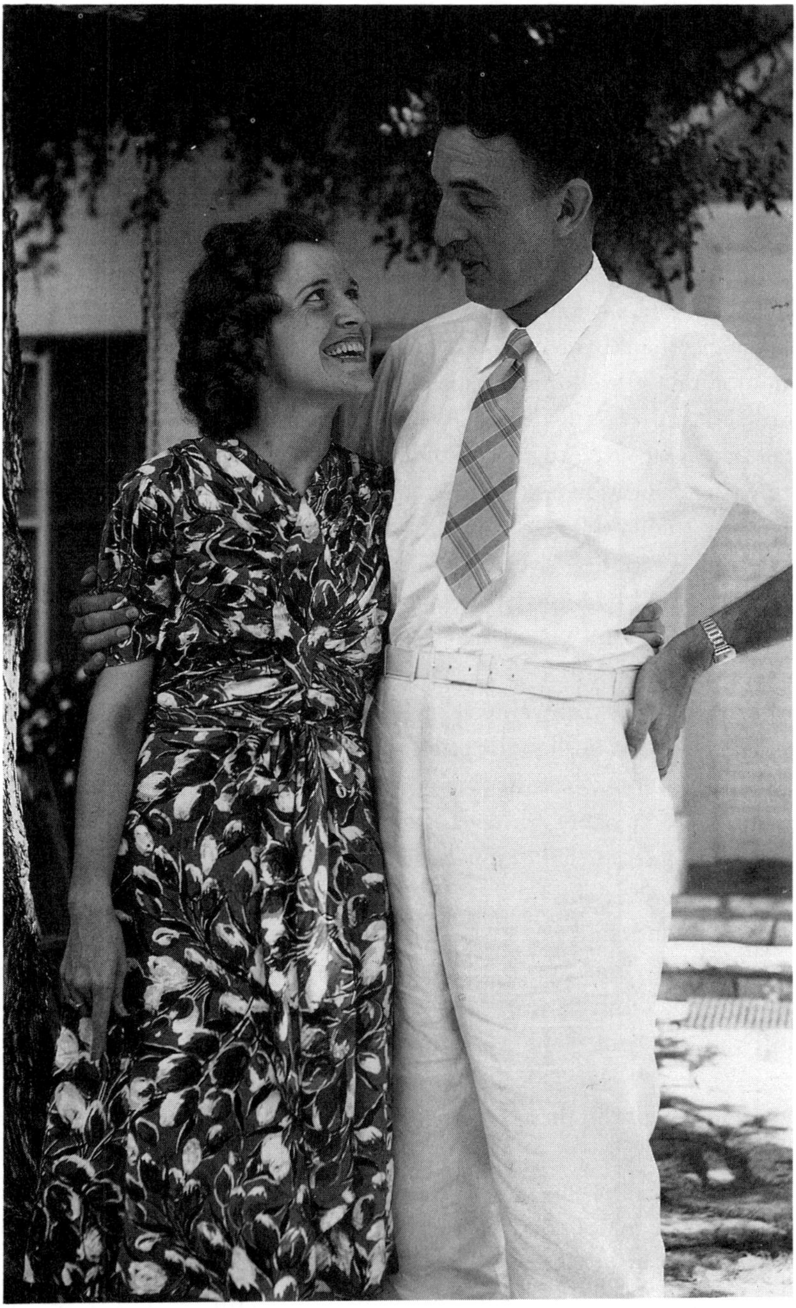

Jim and Edith Cameron on their wedding trip—August 1939.

threshold of the house we lived in down on what is now Elk Parkway overlooking the Tallapoosa River.

The war in Europe started only two weeks later (September 1, 1939), and the world has been upset a great deal since that time.

Mr. Tom Russell had the upstairs of the house at Lake Hills converted from an attic to a sitting room, a bedroom, and a bath. Edith and I lived upstairs, and Granny lived downstairs in that house for several months. In about October of 1940, my friend Dr. Ernest Askin was called up for active military duty and left a little house on South Central Avenue. When that happened, we rented the house from Bragg Comer, and Granny moved into an apartment in the same neighborhood. The little house on South Central Avenue was within a nine-iron shot of the railroad, very close to the hospital, and close to town. It was a most convenient location and a happy place too.

On July 21, 1941, our first child, Edith (Chick), was born at Russell Hospital. Edith had a very severe complication of pregnancy known as eclampsia and had a narrow escape from dying. Chick weighed seven pounds, two ounces and had nearly a thousand pounds of doctors looking after her mother. That was the beginning of our family.

Chick was a very wanted child. We had been on pins and needles for a couple of years until we had a baby. We just knew we weren't going to have any children because we had been married for two years, but we finally had us a baby. Edith was very disappointed when the doctor told her it was just one child, not twins. She wonders now what she would have done with twins.

That one child was a typical old folks' family. After all, I was an old man of thirty-four, and Edith was twenty-seven when Chick was born. But then a couple of years later we had Elaine (Laney), and Laney was different. She ruled the roost in many ways from her birth on. Only thirteen months later Eleanor was born. Our only son, Jimmy, was born in 1948. Finally, in the spring of 1951, Elizabeth was born; however, she lasted only three months before she died suddenly for no explainable reason, and Jimmy died in 1984 of melanoma. Thus we were blessed with a house full of children after we thought we weren't going to have any. They were all different from each other. Luckily, we frequently get to see the three girls who survive—sometimes all three in one day. They all live here in this little town with us. We feel that we are the most blessed

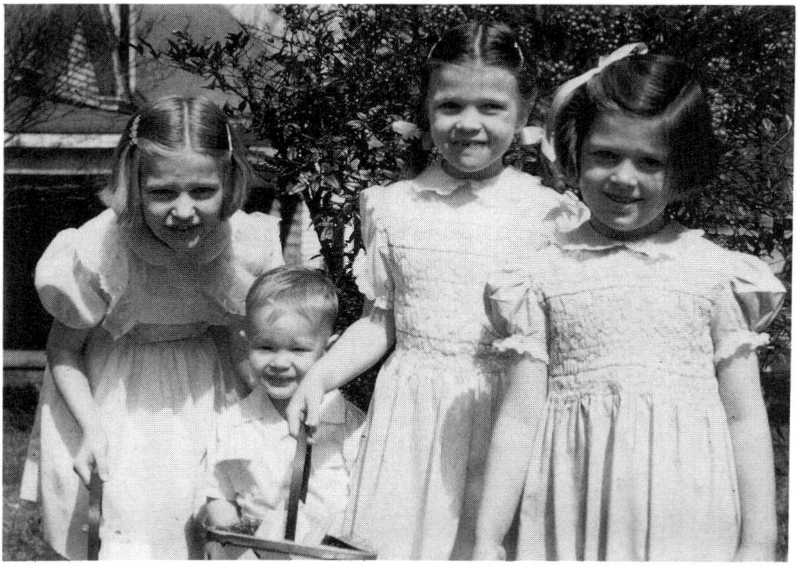

The Cameron children in 1950: Edith, Jimmy, Elaine, and Eleanor.

people at all by our girls living here so near to us. We have friends whose children are scattered out from one state to another, and they are very envious of us.

In the summer of 1943, we had moved from the little house on South Central Avenue to a larger house at 405 Greene Street. This house belonged to the family of Mr. Johnny Carlisle. Mr. Carlisle had died, and his wife lived with a daughter in Eclectic, but the children wouldn't consent to sell the house during their mother's lifetime. However, they did lease it to us. During the time we leased it, we had extensive work done on it including installation of a coal-burning furnace, rewiring, insulation, and a second bathroom. A couple of years later, Mrs. Carlisle died, and her heirs decided to sell the house. The first we knew that they wanted to sell it was when Edith's cousin, Joe Sneed, came down to look at it with the idea of buying it for his family. Since we had a vested interest in the house, we got in the bidding too and did buy it for the then princely price of $7,200.

It was certainly not a new house, having been built soon after the big fire of 1902. Dee Graves, who was approximately my age, was born in that house, but his parents had later built another house next door. Behind the house were Mr. Graves's garden, a smoke house, and a barn. One of the first things we did after we bought the house was to tear down the old barn and smoke house. But when we did that, our house was invaded by large rats! With the help of my friend Dr. Miller, who was a veterinarian, we got rid of the rats, but they were a real hazard for a while.

Incidentally, Pa Graves, (W. D. Graves, Sr.) had had a checkered career. At one time or another he had been a steamboat captain, a diamond merchant, a money lender, and a farmer. He was also a well-educated man. He and another fellow had once spent a summer in Europe when that was not at all common. They had gone from capital to capital by steamboat and railroad.

Around Alexander City in the 1940s, there was no land available on which to build a nice house. No real estate agent had developed any lots in many years. So Dr. Miller and I decided we would like to have some land to build on. We talked to Smith Wilbanks who owned a hundred acres which seemed desirable, but he didn't want to sell it. Bennie Russell also was interested in building a home, so he went to Mr. Wilbanks and convinced him to sell the land to him. Bennie kept enough to build himself a home, and then he agreed to sell the rest to us. His two lots are the two between the highway (old U. S. 280) and the rest of the houses on Ridgeway Drive. He built a lake on his property, but he died before he progressed any further. Then World War II came along and post-poned our plans for several years.

Four of us (Jesse Miller, Ralph Frohsin, Sam Bradshaw, and I) paid Bennie Russell's widow for the land which became Ridgewood Subdivision. Edith Russell had insisted that we take in Sam Bradshaw as a partner before she would sell Bennie's part. We were never sorry to have Sam as a partner, but Ralph, Jessie, and I had laid all the plans before Sam became involved. We tried very hard to do everything right as far as the law, engineering, and layout were concerned. We hired a landscape architect to lay off the lots and price them. There were also certain restrictions drawn up, but these only lasted for twenty-five or thirty years by law. At the end of that time, they were renewed by the consent of every lot owner.

The first houses which were built were those around the circle in Meadowbrook. They were built as soon as the war was over. We got permission from the government to build houses down there to be used by returning soldiers, and those ten or fifteen houses were sold before they were completed. Then, after we four developers drew straws and chose the lots we wanted, we sold off the other lots. The house built by the James Callahans, now owned by Melba Mayfield, was the first house built after those in Meadowbrook. We began our house in 1950 and moved into it in January 1951. The Frohsins and Bradshaws built about the same time, but Dr. Miller never built there.

When our children grew old enough to travel with us, we took them around to the four corners of the United States as then defined; Alaska and Hawaii had not yet become states. We went to the northwest corner of Washington state, the southwest corner of California, the southernmost tip of Florida, and even out to the end of Maine near Calais. In all we traveled to almost all the forty-eight states, across the southern rim of Canada, and into northern Mexico. Thus we traveled rather extensively with our kids and had a good time doing it.

When I first came to Alexander City, my only relative in town was my grandmother. What little family I had lived elsewhere. Now I am kin or kin by marriage to half the people in town because my three daughters

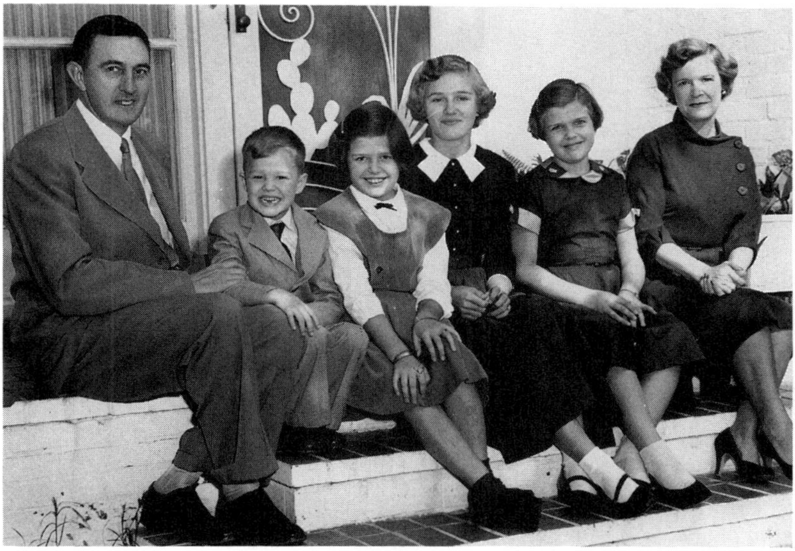

The Cameron family at their Ridgeway Drive home—1954. (The children are, from left, Jimmy, Eleanor, Chick, and Laney.)

all married local fellows (Freddie Blankenship, Russell Mayfield, and David Carlisle) from big families. That made me mahooten (the Jewish word for the parents of those one's children marry) to many people. Furthermore, some of our grandchildren have married into other large local families (Daughertys, Gwaltneys, Holleys, and Guys). And when our family gets together now for Christmas or other holidays, we number thirty-six and we're still growing. Of our ten grandchildren, seven live in Alexander City, and seven of our nine great-grandchildren also live here. All of those who can talk call me "Boompa." [*See* Appendix for complete list of family members.]

My nickname "Boompa," originated when Chick and her husband Freddie went to see a movie starring Jimmy Stewart called "Mr. Hobbs Takes a Vacation." In this movie there was a little boy about three years old who was "in the objective case." When anybody said anything about his grandfather, whom he called "Boompa," he spoke up and said, "I hate

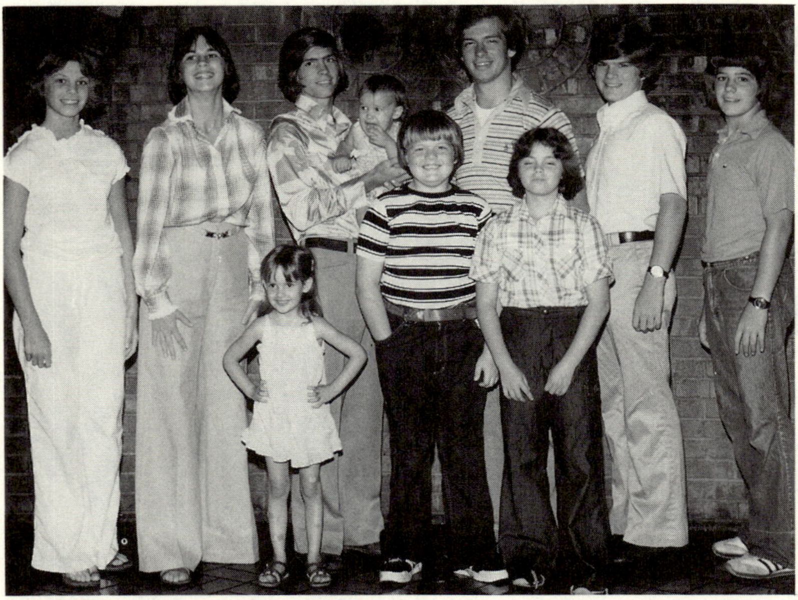

The Cameron grandchildren in 1978—Elaine Mayfield, Ellison Mayfield, Ashley Cameron, David Blankenship holding Angela Cameron, David Carlisle Jr., Martin Blankenship, Cameron Carlisle, Joe Blankenship, and Alfred Blankenship.

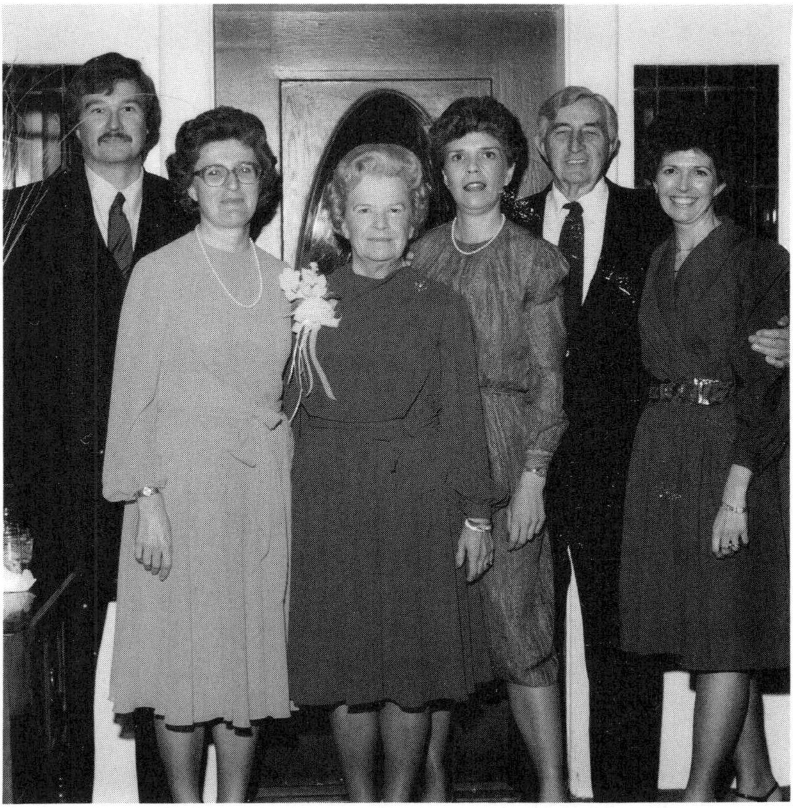

Dr. and Mrs. Cameron and their children—January 1984: Jimmy Cameron, Edith Cameron Blankenship, Edith E. Cameron, Elaine Cameron Mayfield, Dr. Cameron, Eleanor Cameron Carlisle.

Boompa!" This was because Boompa made him mind, in contrast to his very permissive parents. This movie came out about the same time that our first grandchild, David Blankenship, was a baby, and because several things about the movie reminded Chick and Freddie of our family, they decided that I should be called Boompa. And now, not only our grandchildren but many of the friends of our children and grandchildren, such as the Dobbs, Parks, Crowes, Blythes, Denneys, Mayfields, and Wolfes, also use this name which is a term of endearment as far as I am concerned.

14

Boy Scouts and Drunk Masons

DURING THE EARLY 1940S, I WAS THE LEADER OF an Explorer Boy Scout Troop. In that group were Jack White, Robert White, Gene Wolfe, Myron Sasser, Junior Hall, Henry Willis, James Earnhardt, and some other fine young men. We met in the basement of the Alexander City Bank building. During the war, one of our activities was a course in aircraft recognition. Thus if a bomber came over, we would be able to recognize friendly as well as enemy aircraft. Another project was building and flying of model airplanes. Most of the boys stayed in the group until they were either drafted, went to college, or were eighteen years old.

When I was still a rather young man, in 1948, I was elected to the city council. I served for four years. Council members in those days were paid only a pittance. I was happy to serve my city, but I did not choose to run for re-election. Now some council members call themselves making politics a way of life; if they get elected to the city council, they want to be re-elected for life. But I don't believe that's they way things ought to be.

The biggest project I was involved in with the Chamber of Commerce was the erection of local schools, both the Benjamin Russell High School and Laurel High School. Several of us went around and begged money for Benjamin Russell High School with the promise that no federal or state money would be used in the project. Thus it would be a purely local project, and the federal government would have no say in what we could and couldn't do. That was a big selling point in getting people to contribute. As soon as Benjamin Russell was completed, we realized that the black children didn't have an equally good high school, so with some reluctance we convinced people to finance a black school under the same stipulations. Of course, those stipulations have long since gone by the wayside.

I was also active for a number of years in the Lions Club. Our main project was furnishing uniforms and instruments for the high school band. The band was the Lions Club's "baby," and we sold concessions at the football games and had softball games, minstrels, and all kinds of other activities to raise money for the band. In the end it would have been easier for each of the hundred or so members of the club to give ten dollars than to sell tickets to all those fund-raising activities.

I took up Masonry because my brothers-in-law Frank and Herman Ellison were involved in the Masons and highly recommended it. However, I found it was very unsatisfactory to attend a meeting and be called out to attend the sick. These calls disturbed the whole meeting. I did remain in this organization long enough to attain the degrees which qualified me to go to the Shrine in Montgomery. I decided that Shriners were just drunk Masons.

15

Radio, Flying and Snake Killing

DURING MY LIFE I HAVE ENJOYED MANY HOBBIES, probably more than I should have. One way or another, I have fooled with ham radio since 1916. In 1916, my across-the-road neighbor, Bergen Hawkins, had a "wireless" which occupied a space of several square feet and put out maybe one-fourth of a watt of power with which he could talk to his neighbor who lived up the street using Morse code. I frequently went over to Bergen's house and played with him and his wireless. At nine o'clock each night amateur operators listened intently for the time signal sent out from Arlington, Virginia, so that ships at sea could set their chronometers. Every Saturday we would take the antenna down and polish the wire, thinking it would get a little more radiation. There was no such thing as vacuum tubes in those days, so his receiver was a crystal receiver.

In the spring of 1917 the United States got into World War I, and the amateur radio operators in America had to literally destroy their apparatus and suspend all activity until 1919.

In 1921 was the first broadcast of any sort in the United States. By that time Deforest had invented the vacuum tube. One day at school a boy came and told me that he had heard on the wireless the night before that Harding had been elected President. The boy was a notorious fib teller, so I questioned his story. Then he invited me out to his house that evening to hear the wireless. I went to his house in a suburb of Birmingham near where I lived, and we heard a man playing "Ten Little

Fingers and Ten Little Toes." Of course we had on headphones. I immediately went outside to see where the Victrola was set up, but there was none. The man on the wireless said he was at KDKA, the Westinghouse Electric and Manufacturing Co. in East Pittsburgh, Pennsylvania. He wanted everyone who heard him to write or give him a call telling on what frequency and at what time they had heard what tune. He promised to correspond with them later. And that was my introduction to radio broadcast. I went home and started building myself a set the next day. I continued to play with radio for a while until my interest waned.

Along about 1933, I decided to try radio again and made an attempt to learn code. I bought a small receiver with one tube, but I soon aborted that attempt because of my medical practice in Eclectic.

Thus it was 1960 before I managed to get a license and operate my own ham radio. I have played with ham radio ever since then. I have "worked" all states including Hawaii and Alaska (before they became states) and have cards confirming these conversations as well as those from about seventy-five to one hundred foreign countries. I received an award from the American Radio Relay League for having WAS (worked all states). I have talked to both poles, all continents, and all seas. At the present time I have a transmitter and receiver which enable me to talk in sideband, fm, am, and all modes. The amplifier that I had with the set I bought in 1963 is still workable, though not connected. Though the Collins gear I bought in 1963 was the very best available then, I had to modernize when the vacuum tube became hard to get. The apparatus I have now is all transistorized and is very much better than the old tube variety. I can use a maximum of one hundred watts power which is very satisfactory. I also have a two-meter rig.

Radio has been a life-saving hobby for me. I thoroughly enjoy communicating with other people both far and near. One of my most satisfying experiences was when I was able to connect a local woman, Ruth Harwell, with her son Thomas at the South Pole. He was at the geographic South Pole, not at Little America, when I arranged for his mother to talk to him.

I have also talked with many ships at sea. Incidentally, I talked to the Queen Mary on her last day at sea, before she came into Long Beach, California as a permanent exhibit. I once talked to a man and his son in Wales who had only a two-watt transmitter, but atmospheric conditions and sunspot activity were such that I was able to have solid conversation with them.

I have even visited with a man met through radio named Hans Jungdahl who lived near the town of Ribe in Denmark. Edith and I went by and had lunch with him and his family and took his children some music on tapes. I had asked him what I might bring when I came; he said his little girls were crazy about taped music, so I took tapes of "My Fair Lady," "Fiddler on the Roof," and some other good music. However, when I got to Denmark and asked these twelve-to-fifteen-year-old girls

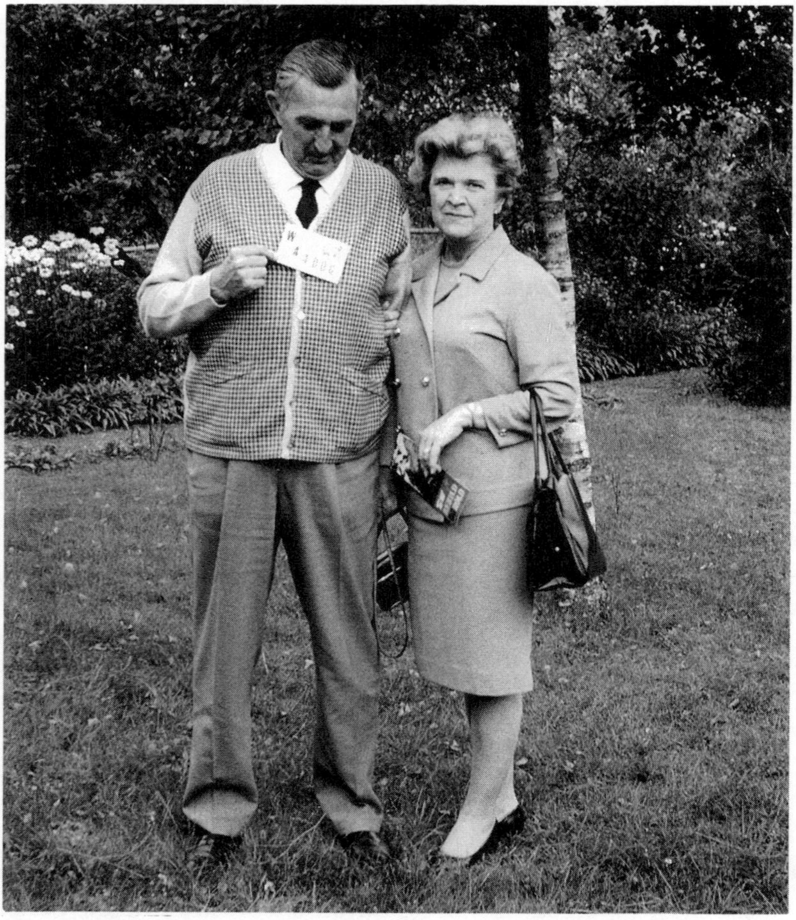

Jim and Edith Cameron in Denmark at the home of Hans Jungdahl, a Dane whom Jim "met" through ham radio—1967.

what kind of music they liked best, they said, "Country and western music! Johnny Cash is our favorite artist." So they weren't much different from the teenagers back home.

I have really had a good time talking to people around the world. Of course, I don't speak any language except English and a few words of Spanish, but between the two I manage to get along pretty well communicating with people.

Besides amateur radio, airplanes have fascinated me most of my life. Having been born in 1907, I was around for the first stages of air travel. The Wright brothers had first flown a controllable aircraft in 1903 though there had been balloon flight many years earlier.

During World War I, aircraft had been used in battle and reconnaissance. In 1919 there were aircraft everywhere and the advent of great flying was upon us. Into Birmingham that year came a man named Eddie Stinson and his sister Catherine Stinson who had operated a flying school teaching soldiers to fly during the first World War. Eddie Stinson had been the first man to solve the mystery of the spin, the result of the plane stalling; up until his day the spin had usually been fatal. Stinson discovered that by pushing the stick forward and making the plane go faster, the pilot could usually regain control in time to avoid a crash.

The first time I got a chance to ride in an airplane was in January 1919. During the Christmas holidays, I had worked at the Butcher Tool and Hardware Co. and made five dollars per day. The owner was a friend of my stepfather, and thus at age eleven I had obtained this temporary job. Anyway I had saved my money, and it was burning a hole in my pocket. When I found I could pay for a ride in a Curtis Oriole airplane on a Sunday in the middle of January, I went out to Dixie Flying Field (near Elmwood Cemetery) and for ten dollars bought a ride from Eddie Stinson. This bi-plane had a six-cylinder engine upright and in-line. The radiator sat between the wings right in front of the pilot. The pilot sat behind the double passenger seat. The Oriole was the latest thing in airplanes and probably cost five thousand dollars.

We took the plane to the end of the field followed by two men on a motorcycle who helped turn the plane into the wind. Eddie gave it the gun, and we took off. After we had flown around the field for a few minutes, Eddie decided to do some acrobatics to draw a crowd and get some more suckers to pay ten dollars for a ride. He did a couple of loops and other maneuvers, and then we landed. Well, I was thrilled no end! I even took some pictures with my Brownie Kodak of the plane I had ridden in that day.

From then on I had the itch and wanted to fly every chance I got. I did get one more chance for two dollars. When I was in Tuscaloosa, about 1924 or 1925, I rode in an Eaglerock bi-plane. The first time I rode in a commercial plane was in 1931 when I rode from Birmingham to Dallas, Texas. This plane was a Fokker tri-motor which carried about fourteen passengers and had wicker seats in it.

As we were flying along at about two thousand feet, the co-pilot came back to inform the passengers we would stop at Meridian, Mississippi, to refuel and get lunch. He told us what our options were for lunch, then went back to the cabin and in Morse code communicated our orders to the ground. When we landed at Meridian after a flight of about two hours, we went into a shed and ate while the airport crew refueled the plane. We thought that was really marvelous advancement in flying.

I didn't learn to fly an airplane until during World War II when everybody wanted to learn to fly. There were a few doctors then who flew small planes which would carry one patient on a stretcher. This type of flight was used only in close support of military action in isolated spots in the world. But I had visions of learning to fly that kind of plane.

The plane I did actually learn to fly was a forty-horsepower cub with no tail wheel, brakes, or electrical system. The engine had a single ignition system, not the dual ignition system which came later. The big forty-horsepower engine would get the plane off the ground in no wind in only perhaps one thousand feet. One had to fly from Alexander City nearly to Lake Martin to get up to two thousand feet. The plane took off and landed at about thirty-five mph and cruised at about sixty-five mph. Planes had a very limited gasoline supply, so the maximum altitude was about fifteen thousand feet on a good clear day. But it was quite a lark to get to fly.

The expense of flying in those days was not great. The plane initially cost less than one thousand dollars. Fuel cost approximately twenty-five cents per gallon, and the plane burned about four gallons per hour.

Few people were qualified as flight instructors—some civilian and some military. My first instructor was an army man who, along with his wife, was later killed in Texas when their car was caught in a flash flood.

Then I had an instructor named Jack Williams from Anniston, Alabama. Jack flew with me until I soloed after about eight hours of instruction. When he got out of the airplane, it behaved entirely differently from the way it had with him in it. So on my first solo flight, I had a hard time getting the plane back on the ground; it wanted to take off sooner than I expected and to keep flying because it was so much lighter than it had been with the two of us in it.

Darwin Dobbs had bought a plane in about 1942 or 1943. This was a Funk airplane, a no-nonsense plane with side-by-side seating and a 63-horsepower Ford Model-B engine turned upside down and backward. Where the clutch plate had been, the propeller was bolted on. Where it had had a splash oil system, it had an oil pump, a sump pump, and an oil reservoir. The pilot had to open and close doors to let air in to the radiator to regulate the temperature. This was really a hybrid, half automobile and half airplane, but it flew very well. Very few people were ever hurt in a Funk. It was spin resistant, not spin-proof, but you did have to try hard to make it spin, and it wanted to come out of a spin by itself.

One of the nicest things about this plane was that you could pull the wheel back into your lap to bring the plane into a stall, yet the plane would go straight ahead, not fall off into a spin. It would also lose altitude very rapidly. So if you wanted to come in over a field and land short, you pulled the wheel back into your lap and the plane went down like an elevator. Just when you got down to about two hundred feet, you pushed the control forward to pick up speed and landed, a rather unique landing system.

The Funk had brakes, a tail wheel, and wheel pants—very advanced features for that time.

First and last, I have had many flying experiences. I flew the Funk all over the southern United States. Then I had a Cessna 140, the Silver Bullet, which I flew to Chicago, New York, Atlantic City, North Carolina a few times, and to Florida a couple of times. I took Jimmy to Sebring, Florida, to the races in the Silver Bullet on his eighteenth birthday.

In 1969, my son-in-law Freddie Blankenship, Bill Byrd, and I pooled our resources and bought a Cessna 185, a Skylane (N1970-X), a four-place plane large enough inside for front and back seat passengers to exchange places in flight, which wasn't true of any other small plane I knew of. It had a 225-horsepower engine and a cruising range of some seven hundred plus miles. It was so satisfactory we flew it all around. Freddie, Edith, and their children flew it to Maine and eastern Canada; we also flew it to Miami. Skylanes are still for sale though they are no longer made. This plane had fixed landing gear, a controllable speed propeller, flaps, and a full panel of the latest navigational devices including twin omnis. It was quite an advancement over my earlier planes. When we sold this plane in about 1972 or 1973, we got as much for it as we had paid for it a few years earlier.

Though I had flown for about thirty years, from the 1940s to the 1970s, I had never gotten an instrument rating. I had flown by the seat of my pants and looking at a regional or aerial map. Then I decided I wanted to learn to fly better, so I took a course in instrument flight. My instructor was Carmen Turner, the Russell Company pilot and a very understanding and thoughtful man. He instructed me in the seventies early in the mornings in all kinds of weather over a period of about six months. I had to have a certain number of hours in instrument flying instruction as well as instruction in map reading and all aspects of flight planning for a most difficult eight-hour written examination.

The first time I took the written exam in Birmingham, I did not pass it. Then I got some additional instructional manuals, studied some more, and passed the test when I took it again. But it was very hard. I went to Monroeville, Alabama, to take the flight section of the test from an instructor who was a perfect stranger to me. I did pass this test, yet I never felt that I was a really competent instrument pilot. I wanted to be able to get out of tight places such as sudden bad weather and adverse circumstances and perhaps do a little night flying. I did do that, but I never felt like I should take off into known icing conditions or other bad weather like some pilots do. However, I did feel that I could probably manage to extricate myself if I were trapped in a bad situation.

All in all, I built model airplanes and flew small airplanes many times for about forty years.

Before I married, the gold mine at Hog Mountain (a few miles from Alexander City) was in full swing. I had two young friends, Neil Johnson and E. J. Alderfer, who were engineers at the gold mine. John Coley, who was also unmarried, was teaching school here then. All of us loved to play bridge, so John and I would call Johnson and Alderfer and get them to come down with some of their nuggets and we'd play bridge all Saturday afternoon, Saturday night and Sunday. John was a much better player than the rest of us, so thanks to John's skill, he and I would take all the gold off the other two. Sometimes we might win as much as twenty dollars, and we had a great time. That was about 1936 or 1937, so I have been playing bridge a good long while though I was never an expert, never as good as my wife.

In addition to the sailboat which I built in Eclectic, I built a cabin cruiser in 1948, the same year Jimmy was born. This boat took about two years to build, but on it and other boats I have been on all the rivers in Alabama from east to west and north to south. Boating has not been a major hobby with me though I also sailed some. Jimmy had a sailboat for several years, and he and I once sailed from Pensacola to Naples, Florida, a distance of about seven hundred miles.

Once when my son Jimmy was a boy, he and I put a canoe into the Tallapoosa River at Wadley, Alabama. We got well down into Tallapoosa County and were overturned by a tree that had fallen into the river. We managed to get out of the river but had to walk a long way to find someone to help us free our canoe and give us a ride back home. That pretty well ended our canoeing days.

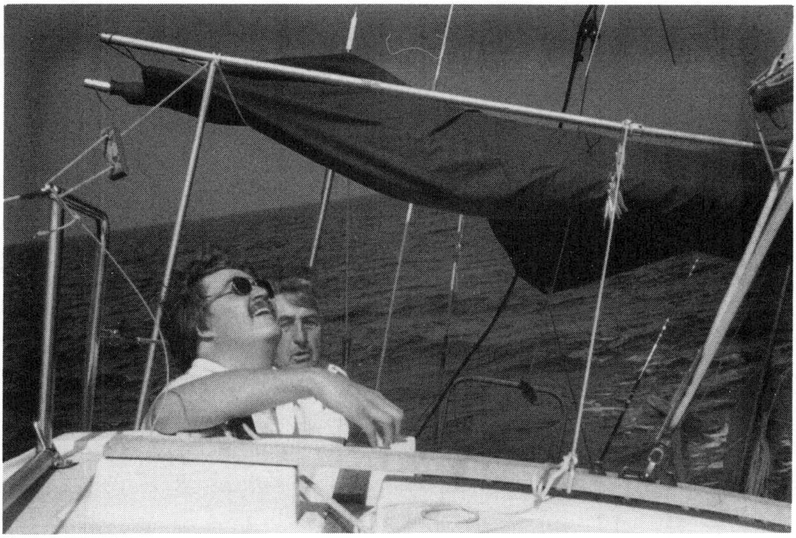

Jimmy and Jim Cameron on the Prime Rate *in the Gulf of Mexico—1980.*

I have tried many sports and excelled at none. I have tried skeet shooting and golf in eleven different countries. I still missed short putts and hooked my drives, no matter what country I was in. Golf has been a prominent time waster for me.

One amusing incident related to golf occurred about 1935 as Jim Farrior and I were going to Panama City. Our old buddy "Hog" Roberts had arranged for us to play golf at the Panama City Country Club, but he was not able to play with us because he had a baby case at the moment. Thus we were paired with two strangers from New York who were much better golfer than Farrior and I. They tried to get us into a sizable bet in which we had no interest. But they were beating us handily until about the third hole. On that hole, Farrior saw a small, harmless snake running across the course. He took out his nine iron and cut the snake's head off. Well, when one of the city boys saw what he had done, he said, "Wasn't that a snake you killed?"

"Yeah, haven't you killed any yet? There are lots of them out here."

From then on we had no trouble handling that pair of Yankees. They were busy looking for snakes instead of playing golf.

Much later I was reminded of this incident when I had the pleasure of entertaining one of my former professors on the golf course at Willow Point. This man was a professor of medicine at the University of Utah and was visiting Dr. Tinsley Harrison. Dr. Harrison had invited Edith and me to play golf with the doctor and his wife. As we were playing hole number five, a snake about ten inches long ran across the course. Since the visitor was nearest the snake, I suggested he take his nine iron and cut off the snake's head. He struck at the snake a couple of times and jumped back as if he were frightened. So I asked if he were afraid of the little snake. Then he confessed that that was the first time he had ever seen a live snake outside a zoo. Now this man was world-famous and had lectured all over the world, yet he was afraid of a snake about ten inches long.

I got my first dose of gardening during the fifth grade in school when our principal had us spade up a garden near the school yard. The principal tried to teach us what the numbers on fertilizer sacks meant and how things grew through germination and cross-pollination, but I didn't really get into gardening until our friend Gordon Taylor kept bringing us produce from his garden. I was embarrassed to keep taking his produce

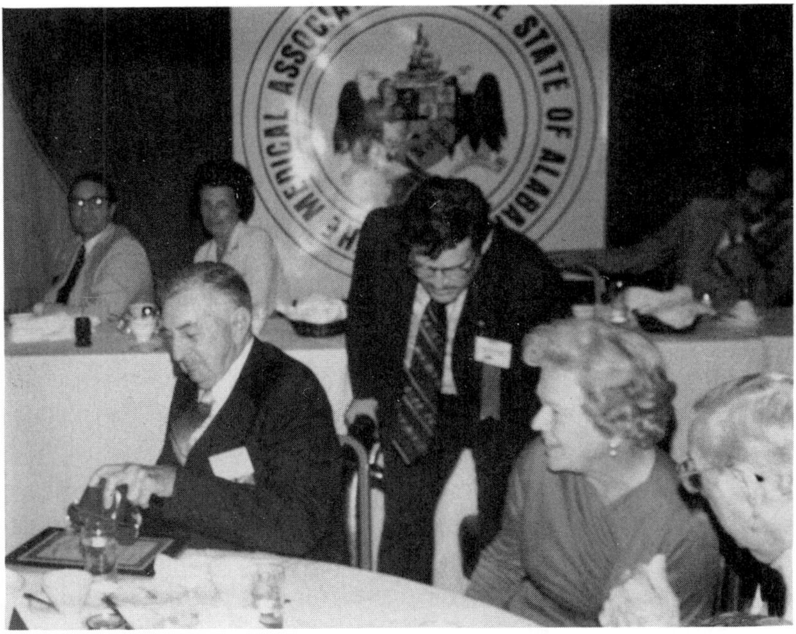

Dr. Cameron is recognized by the Medical Association of Alabama for his fifty years of practice—1980.

and not produce some of my own, so about the time I retired, I began gardening on my own a little bit. However, I was never an avid gardener.

Edith and I have traveled somewhat. We have been to Europe several times and particularly like Scotland and Denmark. We have played golf in Scotland and Denmark five or six times and traveled more extensively in Denmark than we have in Alabama.

More recently we have cruised through the Panama Canal. We also made one trip to the eastern part of the Mediterranean, the Holy Land, and Asia Minor. A few years ago we also went to Alaska. The last cruise we went on, in the Baltic Sea, was on a very small ship where we were able to move around better than on a larger ship. It only had two hundred passengers in contrast to some ships which carry two thousand passengers or more. So we haven't exactly stayed at home all the time, and there are some things we need to do yet, including going on another cruise if possible.

I love to read as well as play with my ham radio, so I'm not in too bad a shape for an old man. I love to read almost anything except what somebody told me I had to read or what I felt naturally compelled to read. Such things as Gibbon's *Decline and Fall of the Roman Empire*, Prescott's *History of the Conquest of Mexico*, H. G. Wells's *Outline of History* were things I felt compelled to read. I would say that my favorite type of book is the historical novel. I certainly read a great deal during the year I lay on my back in a hospital recovering from tuberculosis, and I still read several books at a time. Winston Churchill is definitely my favorite author.

My wife is much more active physically than I am. She's just a girl of eighty-one while I am an old man of eighty-seven and a half. As a matter of pride, she doesn't like being reminded that she's in her eighties.

I retired from the practice of medicine in 1982 after having treated sick folks for fifty-two plus years. I hung up my shingle and have treated no people since that time. But the grateful patients whom I see in the grocery store and other places make me happy that I did try to treat sick people, and some of them got well in spite of it.

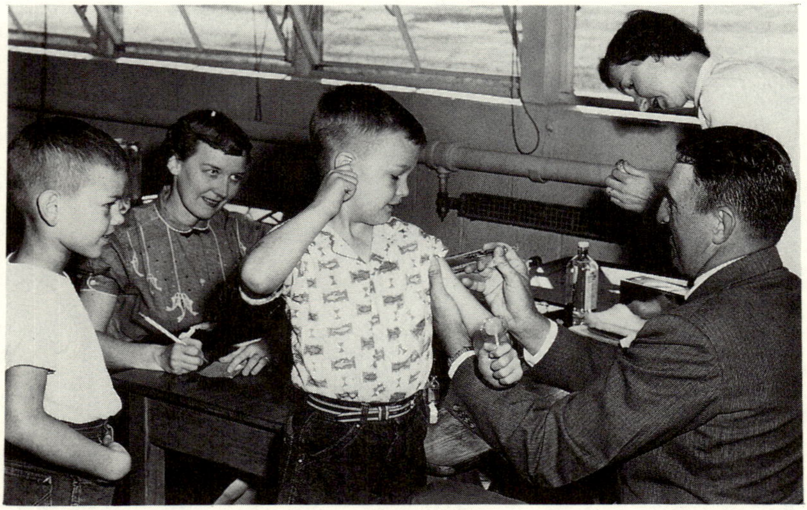

Dr. Cameron gives polio vaccine to his son Jimmy (as well as other first graders)—April 1955.

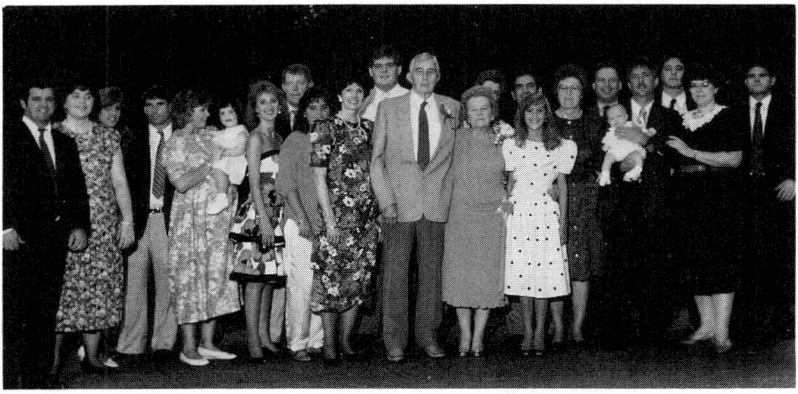

Cameron family, July 30, 1989, at Dr. and Mrs. Cameron's fiftieth wedding anniversary:
(L-R) Randy Holley, Ellison Mayfield Holley, Ashley Cameron, Gene Gwaltney, Elaine Mayfield Gwaltney, Caroline Gwaltney, Scooter Cameron, David Carlisle Sr., Cameron Carlisle, Eleanor Cameron Carlisle, David Carlisle Jr., Dr. Jim Cameron, Edith Ellison Cameron, Elaine Cameron Mayfield, Angela Cameron, Freddie Blankenship, Edith Cameron Blankenship, Martin Blankenship, Scott Blankenship held by David Blankenship, Alfred Blankenship, Christy Blankenship, Joe Blankenship.

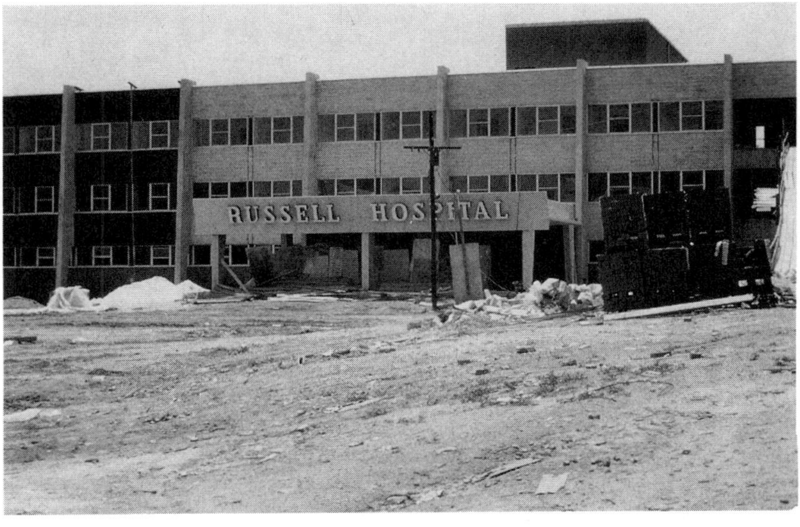

Russell Hospital under construction—1964.

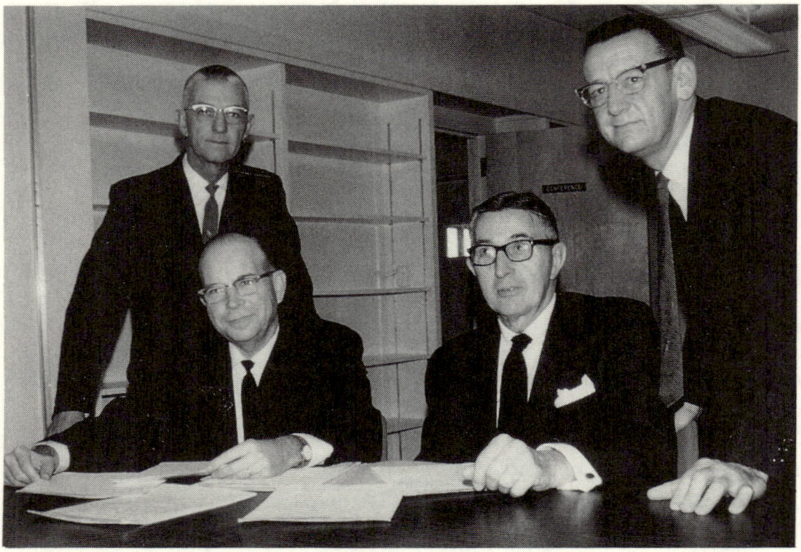

Officers of the medical staff when the new Russell Hospital opened in 1965: (left to right): Dr. Lee Cockerham, secretary; Dr. Ernest Askin, president of the medical staff; Dr. Cameron, vice president of medical staff; Dr. Harold Dark, Chief of Staff.

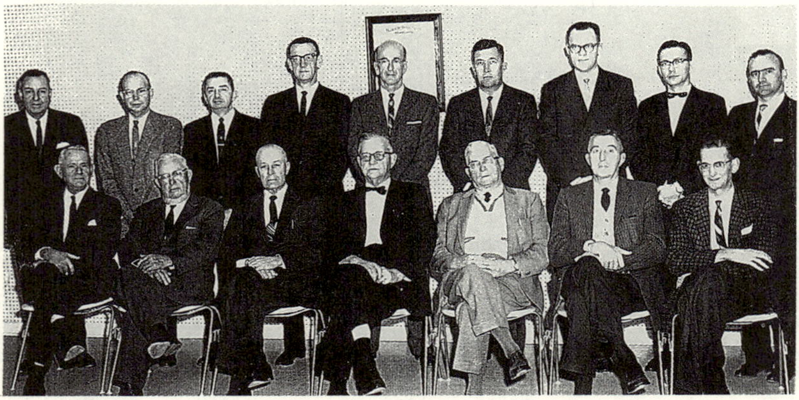

Members of the Tallapoosa County Medical Society in December 1962. (Front, left to right): Dr. Joseph Banks, Dr. J. J. Walls, Dr. Lewis Hamner, Dr. John L. Denney, Dr. R. B. Garlington, Dr. J. E. Cameron, Dr. Lucian Newman. (Back row, left to right): Dr. Wade Lamberth, Dr. H. E. Askin, Dr. John R. Chapman, Dr. Harold U. Dark, Dr. J. H. Harrison, Dr. Lewis Lamberth, Dr. D. E. Owensby, Dr. J. P. Temple, and Dr. A. J. Swindall.

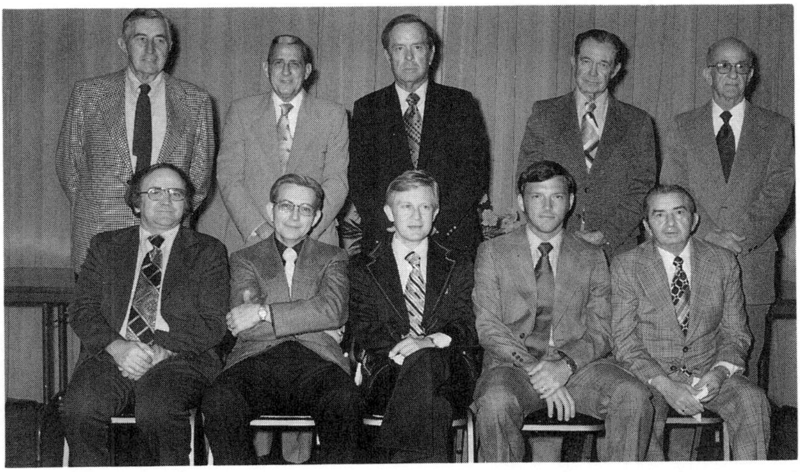

Members of the Tallapoosa County Medical Society (March 1976)—Standing, left to right: Dr. James Cameron, Dr. Robert Heiderpriem, Dr. William Gaba, Dr. Bud Fargason, and Dr. James Harrison. Seated, left to right: Dr. Jerry Swindall, Dr. James Temple, Dr. Joe Stimson, Dr. Vic Hamilton, and Dr. John R. Chapman.

APPENDIX

A. Ancestor Report

B. Descendant Report

C. My Own Medical History

Ancestors of James Edwards CAMERON

Born: 18 Aug 1907, Birmingham, Ala. Married: 1 Aug 1939, Hurtsboro, Ala.

William James CAMERON, Jr.
born: 22 Jul 1881, Birmingham, Ala.
married: 19 Aug 1904, Birmingham, Ala.
died: 21 Oct 1965, Torrance, Calif.

William James CAMERON
born: May 1851, Montgomery, Ala.
married: 12 Dec. 1872, Montgomery, Ala.
died: 27 Nov 1918, Birmingham, Ala.

Andrew CAMERON
born: 1820, County Tyrone, Ireland
married: 1 May 1850, Philadelphia, Pa.
died: 17 Jul 1893, Birmingham, Ala.

Eliza Jane CROZIER
born: 1827, Ireland
died: 10 Jan 1910, Birmingham, Ala.

Mary Elizabeth SMITH
born: 14 Sep 1851, Montgomery, Ala.
died: 2 Aug 1881, Birmingham, Ala.

William Henry SMITH
born: 14 Jun 1814, Suffield, Conn.
married: 23 May 1849, Montgomery, Ala.
died: 25 Feb 1890, Montgomery, Ala.

Julia Pauline HANNON
born: 4 Jun 1831, Knoxville, Crawford Co., Ga.
died: 12 Mar 1885, Montgomery, Ala.

Hallie James EDWARDS
born: 17 Apr 1886, Richmond, Ky.
died: 14 Dec 1922, Asheville, N.C.

Frank Mason EDWARDS
born: Sep 1865, Mississippi
married: 14 Nov 1888, Birmingham, Ala.
died: 16 Sep 1913, Birmingham, Ala.

James F. EDWARDS
died: 1899

Solina A.
died: 26 Jul 1915, Birmingham, Ala.

Virginia "Jennie" McDONALD
born: 17 Aug 1870
died: 26 Feb 1960, Alexander City, Ala.

William McDONALD

Virginia MADISON

The Generations of James Edwards Cameron As Descended from William James Cameron

1 2 3 4 5 6

William James Cameron
b 1851, d 1918, m Mary Booton Ward 1883

William Smith Cameron
b 1874, d 1936, m Mary Frances Harmas 1902, moth. Mary Elizabeth Smith

Clifford Andrew Cameron
b 1902, d 1963, m Madie Lois Jarvis 1923

Madie Lois Cameron
b 1924, m Kenneth Davidson Riley 1992

Harry Clifford Davis
b 1944, father Harry Southerd Davis

Remi Davis
b 1971, mother Marian Wingo

Wade Cameron Davis
b 1973, mother Marian Wingo

Glen Eugene Davis
b 1948, father Harry Southerd Davis

Pauline Cameron
b 1877, d 1974, m Ralph Ussery Falkner 1901, moth. Mary Elizabeth Smith

Andrew Crozier Cameron
b 1879, d 1935, m Louise Harrison 1916, moth. Mary Elizabeth Smith

William James Cameron, Jr.
b 1881, d 1965, m Gertrude Leonard, moth. Mary Elizabeth Smith

Virginia Cameron
b 1905, d 1978, m Emmett Girard Craig 1930, moth. Hallie James Edwards

James Edwards Cameron
b 1907, m Edith Ellison 1939, moth. Hallie James Edwards

Edith Cameron
b 1941, m Freddie Lavelle Blankenship 1960

Martin Luther Blankenship
b 1956

Jesslyn Cameron Blankenship
b 1991, moth. Rebecca Imelda Segars

1 2 3 4 5 6

David Steven Blankenship
b 1961, m Mary Jane Morrison 1994

David Scott Blankenship
b 1989, moth. Chrisleigh Jane Baker

Mallory Elaine Blankenship
b 1991, moth. Chrisleigh Jane Baker

Joseph Cameron Blankenship
b 1963, m Julie Rae Daugherty 1991

Cameron Ray Blankenship
b 1994

Courtney Rae Blankenship
b 1996

Alfred Marion Blankenship
b 1964, m Michelle Elizabeth Lee 1993

Emily Marie Blankenship
b 1995

Elaine Cameron
b 1943, m James Chapman Carlisle 1996

Helen Elaine Mayfield
b 1962, m Eugene Cleveland Gwaltney III 1982, fath. Russell Spenser Mayfield

Caroline Cameron Gwaltney
b 1986

Amelia Staley Gwaltney
b 1989

Edith Ellison Mayfield
b 1963, m Randall Milton Holley 1988, fath. Russell Spenser Mayfield

Eleanor Cameron
b 1944, m Warren David Carlisle 1964

Virginia Cameron Carlisle
b 1968, m Joseph Clayton Guy Jr. 1990

Clayton Carlisle Guy
b 1993

Warren David Carlisle Jr.
b 1970

James Edwards Cameron Jr.
b 1948, d 1984, m Sarah Elizabeth Quick 1970

Ashley Elizabeth Cameron
b 1973

Angela Catherine Cameron
b 1976

1 2 3 4 5 6

Elizabeth Cameron
b 1951, d 1951

George Ward Cameron
b 1887, d 1932

Mary Ward Cameron
b 1889, d 1966, m Yates Wellington Faison 1915

Yates Wellington Faison Jr.
b 1917, m Peggy Rule 1947

Yates Wellington Faison III
b 1947, m Robin Johnston 1994

David Rule Faison
b 1950, m Kim Weller 1978

Christopher Rule Faison
b 1981

Grace McIntosh Faison
b 1983

Jonathan David Faison
b 1985

twins Faison
b 1951, d 1951

Sally Ann Faison
b 1954

William Ward Faison
b 1921

Thad Harrison Faison
b 1957, m Mary Dudley Hanes 1993, moth. Natalie Joy Harrison

Elizabeth Yates Faison
b 1962, m Benjamin David Benson 1995, moth. Natalie Joy Harrison

Cameron Faison
b 1928

Cameron Faison Jr.
b 1958, m Diana Williams 1989, moth. Catherine Stewart

Catherine Carol "Catie" Faison
b 1991

Mary Cameron Faison
b 1993

Mary Stewart Faison
b 1960, m William James Blair III, moth. Catherine Stewart

Mary Cameron Blair
b 1984

1 2 3 4 5 6

Elizabeth Thomas Blair
b 1986

William James Blair IV
b 1988

Catherine Branch Blair
b 1994

Catherine Stewart Faison
b 1962, moth. Catherine Stewart

Catherine Ann Byrum
b 1983

Stewart Gatlin Byrum
b 1985

Margaret Ketchum Cameron
b 1891, d 1971, m Frank Edward Spain 1917

Margaret Cameron (Peggy) Spain
b 1919, d 1996, m William Clifford McDonald Jr. 1944

Margaret Cameron McDonald
b 1947, m John Scott Vowell 1985

John Scott Vowell Jr.
b 1987

William Clifford McDonald III
b 1948, m Nancy Ann Adams 1974

Margaret Ann McDonald
b 1975

Lucy Johnston McDonald
b 1978

William Clifford McDonald IV
b 1983

Frances Edward Spain
b 1922, d 1971, m Jake Chapline Hodges Jr. 1943

Ellen Cameron Hodges
b 1945, m Arthur Powell 1977

Guy Allen Weatherford III
b 1968, d 1991, fath. Guy Allen Weatherford Jr.

Dabney Elizabeth Weatherford
b 1971, fath. Guy Allen Weatherford Jr.

Jake Chapline Hodges III
b 1948, m Peggy Faulkner 1970.

Frank Spain Hodges
b 1973

Justin Michael Hodges
b 1975

Appendix C: My Own Medical History

A Large, 'Knife-Nosed Glaggie'

Having been a doctor all my working life, I have naturally had the most opportunity to observe and monitor my own physical condition.

I was a large baby to whom my mother gave birth apparently without great difficulty. I was an overgrown young child. When I was still in high school, people thought I ought to be in college. And when I was in college, they thought I should have been out. I grew to about six feet, one and one-half inches tall and a maximum weight of about 235 pounds. My fighting weight was about 172, the amount I weighed when I finished medical school.

When I finished medical school, I could lie on my back and in one bound come to a standing position. I was never a very graceful diver, but I was able to do several diving maneuvers.

The hair on my head has always been plentiful; brown for most of my life, it is now gray. My eyes are brown. Now they have arcus senilis, the white ring around the eyes which often comes early in life with a serious illness. People who have a serious illness in their twenties can develop arcus senilis, eyes of old men. My vision is fine; I am still able to read a newspaper without glasses. I do wear glasses from time to time, but I don't wear them for driving and only had to wear them in flying when it was necessary to read a map at night.

The hearing in my right ear is nearly gone, but that in my left ear is still pretty good, especially for lower tones.

My nose has always been a problem to me. I am pinch-nosed or knife-nosed like the Scotsman who was a "knife-nosed glaggie." I guess that would describe my nose which has given me trouble all my life being stopped up and making me a mouth breather for the most part.

My teeth have always been a big problem. They were very uneven with a great overbite. An attempt by an orthodontist to straighten my teeth when I was young was a complete failure. Several of my teeth died in the effort to move them. Somebody else, not me, killed the orthodontist, so I was saved from doing that. Not only were my teeth irregular and protruding but also very soft. I had the advantage of having an excellent dentist when I was an intern, probably the best dentist in Alabama at the time. He put inlays in many of my teeth and did everything he could to save them, but by the time I was thirty-five I had lost practically all of my teeth. The replacements have been so much better than the teeth I grew that I don't see why anybody wants to put up with natural teeth.

The tonsillectomy I had when I was about seven years old started me on a path to much surgery during my life. I have also had hemorroid and hernia operations. I have had several broken bones, including the collarbone, a radius ulna (lower arm bone), toes, nose, fingers, right ankle, and left hip. My bones are not particularly brittle; I just played hard and I think that accounts for my broken bones.

In my old age I am taking medicines to shrink my prostate, lower my blood pressure, and make my heart beat more regularly than it wants to.

In spite of my beginning in a family stricken by tuberculosis, the many broken bones I have had, and my own bout with tuberculosis many years ago, I have enjoyed excellent health for most of my nearly eighty-eight years.

Index